NATURAL BODY BASICS
Making Your Own Cosmetics

by

Dorie Byers

Gooseberry Hill Publications, Inc.
Bargersville, Indiana

Cover photography and author's portrait by Bill Kruger, Carmel, Indiana.

Graphic design by Studio 2D, Champaign, Illinois.

ISBN 0-9652353-0-0
Library of Congress Catalog Card Number 96-94319

First Edition

Dorie would like to hear about your uses of the recipes in this book and about any experimenting that you do with the ingredients she has written about. She can be contacted in care of Gooseberry Hill Publications, Inc., P.O. Box 251, Bargersville, IN 46106.

For additional copies of *Natural Body Basics—Making Your Own Cosmetics*, send inquiries to Gooseberry Hill Publications, Inc. at the above address.

DISCLAIMER

The author and publisher have made every effort to ensure the accuracy and completeness of information in this book. We assume no responsibility for errors, inaccuracies, omissions, or any inconsistency herein.

The safe and proper use of all ingredients and any of the recipes in this book is the sole responsibility of the person(s) using them. The author and publisher are not responsible for any misuse or carelessness by the user. Likewise, the author and publisher are not responsible for any allergic reactions. None of the advice in this book should be mistaken for medical advice. Any concerns about any condition the user may have should be addressed by a professional medical practitioner.

ABOUT THE AUTHOR

Dorie Byers is a registered nurse, substitute teacher, and housewife. She has received her certificate in Master Gardening through the Purdue University Extension Service and has spent many years growing herbs and researching their uses. She also has earned a certificate in Herbal Studies from The School of Herbal Medicine in Suquamish, Washington. She is currently working on studies in herbal medicine through the Herbal Healer Academy in Mt. View, Arkansas. Dorie lives among her herbs in rural southern Indiana with her husband and son.

༄ ༄

Thanks to my husband Rick and son Jason for their help, love, and support. This work wouldn't have been possible if it weren't for you both. Special thanks to Jim for the encouragement. And thanks to Sway, my best tester and critic. I hope you all enjoy my effort. Love to you all.

CONTENTS

⤋ PREFACE ⤋

Taking care of yourself means making choices. We are inundated on a daily basis with ads that tell us we cannot have good skin or beautiful hair without buying and using this product or that one. The fact is, we can attain a healthy appearance without the purchase of these products and be in more control over our well being besides.

Making skin and hair care products out of natural ingredients provides us with an alternative to commercial preparations. A good appearance will be the end result but without unknown chemical compounds and at a great monetary savings.

When reading books and magazine articles with recipes for natural cosmetics I have generally been disappointed by how many of the recipes just don't work. The ingredients don't mix together well and often the consistency isn't pleasing. After researching and trying different ingredients I have come up with many recipes which contain natural ingredients that you can make with a little effort. All the information you need is contained in this book. Read and use it to free yourself from another part of the commercial world.

Here's to your well being!

∾ INTRODUCTION ∾

here are many skin care products available commercially but when you go to the store to make your choice it becomes challenging. Reading the labels only adds to the puzzle. It seems we need a college degree in chemistry to understand the ingredients. We don't actually know what we are putting on our skin and absorbing into our bodies.

Then, the price of these products really amazes me. A tube of good quality hand cream costs from $3 to $12 at a drug or discount store. If the hand cream is purchased at a cosmetics counter in a major department store the price will likely be much higher. Often times the ingredients listed first on these products are water, mineral oil, alcohol, or witch hazel. None of these ingredients are expensive. Alcohol and witch hazel are drying to some skin types, while mineral oil can clog the skin pores. Despite that, these ingredients are common in the majority of skin care products available. Even with the occurrence of a large amount of inexpensive ingredients in these products, the price is still high.

Go to a natural foods store and check out the cosmetics. The ingredients listed on the labels are more understandable in most cases but the price remains expensive. A jar of herbal deodorant cream is $14.95! A tube of face mask costs $11 and the ingredients are clay and a herbal infusion. For the price of the tube of face mask, I could buy a container of clay and a package of dried herbs, make face masks enough to easily last six months, and still have money left over. If the herb I chose to use for the infusion was one I grow, then the price would decrease even more.

Making your own natural cosmetics is not only economical, but is beneficial to your skin. The best part about making your own cosmetics is that with a bit of research and mixing of ingredients available, you can custom-make your products to suit your own skin's needs. You can adjust different natural ingredients to meet your individual requirements and preferences. There are no artificial ingredients, so the mystery and concern of what is being put on your skin and absorbed into your body is absent. It can be a very satisfying activity to make your own body oils, hand creams, and lip glosses. It's as simple as making cookies from scratch. I find I like seeing little jars and pots of creams and powders that I make lined up on the bathroom shelf. I know exactly what is in each container and what it costs to make. I also know what it doesn't have—lots of chemicals with unpronounceable names and a high price tag. It is also very fresh because preparations are mixed as you need them.

Another positive aspect in making your own cosmetics is that you are one step closer to taking responsibility for your own health and well being. You get to choose what you want on your skin, and then you add it to your formula. You cannot be in more control of what you put on your skin than that.

Making your own cosmetics is versatile. Gifts can be individualized for your family and friends, men and women alike. If you know their skin care needs and skin type, you can give a custom made gift. If you don't have that information, make up some fragrant body oil, powder, or soap. That kind of gift is always welcome and the aroma is so much better than the artificial scents added to most products available in stores.

For whatever reason you are making your own cosmetics, it is fun experimenting with all of the ingredients available. Be creative and use the ingredients list, the glossary, and the herb and essential oils sections of this book as your reference guide.

↔ SUPPLIES ↔

*S*pecial supplies aren't required to make cosmetics. Just look in your kitchen cabinets and drawers. Here are the bare-minimum basics:

ESSENTIAL EQUIPMENT

Small to medium saucepan, stainless steel or enamelware

Do not use aluminum saucepans—aluminum cookware can leach into some ingredients and alter them. I make it a point not to use any aluminum cookware for cooking or cosmetics.

Small to medium bowls, heatproof glassware

I usually use heatproof glass measuring cups instead of bowls.

Grater

Don't use your everyday grater—beeswax is nearly impossible to remove. Use an old grater you've picked up at a garage sale.

Measuring cups and spoons

Wire whisk

A smaller size is best, but large ones will work fine.

Rubber spatula

There are new ones of silicone and other new materials that hold up well to heat without becoming brittle that I use in place of rubber ones, but the rubber or plastic ones work fine if you can't find or afford new ones.

Glass jars and bottles

Brown glass is best to prevent ingredients from deteriorating when exposed to light if they are available. Keep, wash, and use extract bottles, baby food jars, and large mouth jars of all kinds. Plastic containers are adequate, but will soak up the odor of anything put in them, and the odor is impossible to eliminate. There are many glass containers that food is packaged in that are very attractive. I have a list of people who save me appropriate containers including the mother of twins who happily passes along baby food jars that would otherwise be thrown away.

Food processor or blender

Whatever you use must be capable of grinding seeds, grains and dried plant matter into very small powder-like particles.

Small to medium sized funnel

Good herb identification book

There are several on the market—go to a book store and browse, or ask a herbalist what they recommend. It must have good descriptions and pictures to make positive identification possible. My favorite is *Rodale's Illustrated Encyclopedia of Herbs* published by Rodale Press. (See bibliography.)

Eye droppers

These are mandatory when working with essential oils. Glass ones are preferable.

SUPPLEMENTAL EQUIPMENT OPTIONS

Double boiler

Enamelware or stainless steel, not aluminum (see note under saucepans). Instead of a double boiler I place a heatproof glass bowl or measuring cup in a saucepan with two to three inches of boiling water in it. This works very well and I have not felt the need to purchase a double boiler.

Mortar and pestle

These can be used to grind or crush herbs or seeds that do not need to be a small powdery size. You can always place whatever it is you want to crush on a cutting board, cover it with plastic wrap, and hit it with a rolling pin if you don't own a mortar and pestle.

Strainer or sieve

A smaller sized one is all you'll need.

⮠ GLOSSARY ⮡

acid mantle – the body fluid that bathes the surface of the skin. It is composed of sweat, fresh sebum and other cell secretions, and is believed to act as a natural defense barrier for the skin.

anti-inflammatory – a substance that works to prevent redness and irritation.

antiseptic – a property that helps to prevent or stop the growth of bacteria.

astringent – a substance that causes the skin pores to tighten, usually temporarily.

cream – an emulsified cosmetic preparation having a thick consistency.

decoction – extracting the properties of a herb by boiling it in water.

dispersible – the ability to be mixed into a substance with even distribution.

emollient – having the property of being soothing or softening to the skin.

emulsifier – a substance that allows oily liquids to be dispersed with non-oily liquids.

extract – a liquid containing the concentrated properties of a herb obtained by a physical or chemical process.

facial steam – placing the face in an enclosed space with steam consisting of boiling water and herbs.

humectant – a substance that promotes the retention of moisture in the skin.

infused oil – oil and selected herbs allowed to steep in sunlight for a given period of time so that the herbal properties are transferred to the oil.

infusion – an introduction of boiling water into a herb to disperse the herbal properties into the water.

lotion – a liquid cosmetic preparation.

macerate – to cause a herb to soften by soaking or steeping.

mask – a cosmetic preparation applied to the face that produces a tightening effect as it dries.

preservative – an additive used to slow decay and spoilage of a mixture.

sebum – a fatty substance secreted by glands in the skin; it has a lubricating quality.

scrub – a coarsely textured mixture gently rubbed on the skin to deeply cleanse.

tincture – a solution of a herbal substance dissolved in alcohol.

tisane – an infusion of herbs and water, similar to a tea.

toner – a substance that when applied to the skin tightens it.

volatile – the ability to vaporize readily.

⤸ INGREDIENTS ⤸

*W*hen buying natural ingredients, pay special attention to the labels on natural oils. Look for cold pressed or low heat processed oils that contain no preservatives and are not extracted with solvents. Oils that will turn rancid quickly and should be purchased in small quantities are wheat germ oil and evening primrose oil.

Almond – A familiar nut used finely ground in facial scrubs.

Aloe Vera Gel – Clear gel from the leaves of the aloe plant. It has healing properties and is used for burns and troubled skin. It also has emollient properties and makes the skin look shiny.

Apricot Kernel Oil – A clear golden colored oil that is useful to soften all skin types and may be used 100% strength on the skin.

Arrowroot Powder – A starch from the root of the arrowroot plant, it can be used in powder mixtures or as a thickener.

Avocado Oil – A golden green very rich oil that absorbs readily. Good for all skin types, especially dry skin. It is effective diluted up to as much as 10%, but can be useful applied full strength. It is one of my favorite oils.

Baking Soda – A powdery white substance with deodorizing properties used in powder mixtures.

Beeswax – A white or golden solid wax made by bees, it is used as an emulsifier and barrier on the skin. Use an old grater to grate and measure. Some companies sell beeswax in "pearl" form that is easier to measure.

Bentonite – A white clay found in the Midwestern United States, it is used in face masks. It turns gel-like when liquid is added.

Borax – A naturally occurring mineral used as an emulsifier and to soften water.

Brewer's Yeast – A by-product of fermented barley used in beer production. It has a very soothing effect on the skin when applied in a mask.

Castile Soap – A soap that contains olive oil or coconut oil as an ingredient. Has a soft foamy lather.

Castor Oil – A heavy clear oil that is softening to the skin and is rarely linked with allergic reactions. It is derived from the beans of the castor plant. It has a distinctive odor and is especially beneficial as an ingredient in diaper creams.

Cellulose Chips – Small pieces of plant derived material that will absorb essential oils and fix them for potpourri or other mixes of dried plant material.

Cocoa Butter – A solid fat derived from cacao beans. It is used on skin to soften and lubricate. A creamy white solid with a chocolate scent, it mixes well with lanolin.

Coconut Oil – A fine moisturizer derived from fresh coconuts. It is a solid to semi-solid white substance when in a container but liquefies on contact with the skin.

Cornmeal – Ground corn used in facial scrubs.

Cornstarch – A white powdery starch from corn. It is used as a powder ingredient or as a thickener.

D-panthenol – A natural occurring form of the B Vitamin pantothenic acid. It is used in shampoo to help hair feel thicker. I have read that there is some evidence that hair absorbs d – panthenol and gives support from within the hair shaft, making it stronger.

Distilled Water – Water purified by a distillation process.

Dried Milk Powder – Dehydrated milk used on skin and in baths to soften.

Essential Oils – Highly concentrated essences of herbs used in very small amounts for aesthetic and/or therapeutic purposes.

Evening Primrose Oil – An oil from the seeds of the evening primrose plant that is used in skin care products. It is often available in gelcaps which can be punctured with a needle and squeezed to release the oil. There is also a liquid form available.

Flaxseeds – Seeds from the flax plant. When soaked, the seeds form a gel used in facial masks.

Fuller's Earth – A naturally occurring clay used in cosmetics and powders. It absorbs moisture including oil.

Grapefruit Seed Extract – A substance extracted from grapefruit seeds using vegetable glycerine. Used in deodorant and skin care products.

Green Clay – From the south of France, this clay is very pure and highly absorbent. Used in masks and powders.

Herbs – Any plant product that has a useful purpose to humans, particularly in a therapeutic way. Can be flowers, leaves, bark, roots, or seeds.

Honey – A sweet product made by bees, it is used as a moisturizer. It is also soothing and healing when applied to troubled skin.

Jojoba Oil – A naturally liquid wax from the jojoba plant, which is found in the desert. It is protective on the skin and has an indefinite shelf life. It helps dry hair hold moisture. It can be used as a natural alternative to petroleum jelly. Another one of my favorites.

Kaolin – Clay used in masks and powders. Also known as white clay.

Lanolin – A natural grease that comes from wool. It is a heavy substance used to protect skin. Some people have a sensitivity to it.

Lemon – The sunny yellow fruit that is useful when added to skin or hair products. It is softening, deodorizing, and lightening.

Liquid Lecithin – A natural substance containing Vitamin E, fatty acids, and minerals. It is used as an emulsifier to blend oil based and water based products. It is also moisturizing. The only form of lecithin used in the recipes in this book is the liquid form.

Oatmeal – The oat grain rolled flat, used in masks and for bathing. It is very soothing to the skin.

Olive Oil – A heavy green gold oil pressed from olives that has a distinctive odor. Can be used full strength on the skin. It is very soothing and softening.

Pure Grain Alcohol – 95% pure alcohol found in liquor stores. It is used to disperse essential oils and herbal essences into other liquids. Not recommended for internal consumption! Substitute good quality vodka if you can't find it anywhere.

Pure Soap – Soap without any additives that can be found in bars or flakes.

Rosehip Seed Oil – Expressed from the seeds of rosehips, it is good for rejuvenating skin and for softening calloused areas. Has a short shelf life—do not buy a lot. It is also good on irritated skin.

Rosewater – Rose scented water that is a by-product of the production of rose essential oil. It is very softening, soothing, and toning to the skin. Smells very good!

Rubbing Alcohol – A poisonous liquid used to disperse herbs or essential oils into other liquids. Not for internal use! Also has astringent and antibacterial properties.

Sea Salt – Coarse salt that is evaporated from sea water and has no minerals artificially added. It contains minerals not found in regular table salt. Used in baths to soften water and draw impurities from the body.

Shea Butter – This comes from the seeds of the Karite tree which is found in Africa. It is very mild, softening, and moisturizing with a rich texture. Comes in a solid form. It makes a smooth consistency in hand creams.

Sunflower Seeds – The seeds of the sunflower are used in masks and facial scrubs. They will become rancid quickly. Store them in the freezer.

Sweet Almond Oil – Derived from sweet almonds, it is a clear pale yellow oil that is well absorbed by the skin. It may be used 100% strength.

Tincture of Benzoin – Benzoin is a resin from an Asian tree in an alcohol based tincture. It is used as a preservative and has deodorizing properties. Not for internal use.

Turkey Red Oil – A specially treated oil used in baths to soften skin because it is water dispersible.

Vegetable Glycerine – A sweet syrupy substance that is a humectant. Used in skin care products. Do not use full strength as it can pull moisture out of your skin.

Vinegar – A sour liquid obtained by acid fermentation of dilute alcoholic fluids. Softens and cleanses the skin and assists in maintaining the skin's acid mantle. Also good on hair as an after shampoo rinse.

Vitamin E – Used in skin care products as a preservative. It comes measured in International Units, or IU. It is often available in gelcaps that can be punctured with a needle and squeezed to obtain the oil. It can also be obtained in a concentrated (32,000 IU per fluid ounce) liquid form that can be measured using an eyedropper. When looking for Vitamin E look for the more concentrated forms so that the amount of liquid used does not interfere with the consistency of the product you are making.

Wheat Germ Oil – A dark golden oil that contains Vitamin E. It has a distinctive odor and heavy feel. Used in skin creams.

Witch Hazel – A distilled fluid of the bark of the witch hazel shrub in an alcohol solution, it is soothing and astringent. Not for internal use.

There is no guarantee that any specific ingredient will not cause a reaction to your skin. Put a small dab of any substance or preparation you have questions about on the inside of your arm and put a bandaid over the spot. Leave this on overnight—if there is no redness or other signs of irritation the next day it should be safe to use.

❧ HERBS ❧

Several years ago a good friend of mine gave me some divisions of herb plants from her garden. Not knowing much about herbs, I bought a good reference book. That was the beginning of my endless curiosity for everything about herbs. At first I was interested in the culinary and decorative properties of herbs. Then, I read more and realized that herbs are old standbys for many modern day substances. Many medicines used by today's medical community are derived from herbs. And, many herbs add a pleasant and therapeutic aspect to making cosmetics and products for the skin. I became intrigued with this idea and studied more. Now, my herb garden has grown from six plants to well over forty and keeps growing as I keep researching all of the uses of different herbs.

Herbs are defined as any plant found useful to man. There are culinary herbs, decorative herbs, herbs for dyeing fabric, herbs for aroma, and herbs for therapeutic uses. Just working with herbs, cultivating, harvesting, and using them is enough to make a person feel good. The scents and sight of these plants are so pleasing. Even plants that we do not normally view as useful gain new respect with varieties of uses from a herbal standpoint, like dandelions and wild yarrow.

If you are going to use herbs fresh, make absolutely sure you have correctly identified the plant. There are several very good herbal reference books available that have pictures of herbs to help you. My favorite is *Rodale's Illustrated Encyclopedia of Herbs*. (See bibliography.) You could find someone well versed in herbs and ask their advice. It is a good idea to read as much as you can on the subject. The more you read, the better your knowledge of herbs will be and the easier it will be for you to experience the usefulness of herbs. In season, visit public gardens with herb beds—this is another good way to see what the real plants look like.

I also want to caution you that herbs can be very powerful when using them. Just because it is a plant doesn't mean that you can use a herb in an unlimited way without researching it. Read and know about each herb that you use. Knowledge is power and moderation in all things, including herbs, is the wise way to go.

There are several herbs I have incorporated into the formulas in this book. Many have been used in the form of an essential oil, which I will cover in a later section. The herbs I have used in their pure state are listed here with a brief explanation of each as it is used in this book.

Basil – This well-known herb is not just for spaghetti sauce—it is useful in infusions for facial care.

Calendula – This flower is also known as pot marigold. The petals of the flower are used. It has the reputation for being soothing and healing. I like to use it in hair rinses, infused oils, and hand creams.

Catnip – No, this herb will not make you roll around in ecstasy like our feline friends do, but the aroma is pleasant and will help lull you to sleep as an ingredient in a sleep pillow.

Chamomile – Fruity scented flowers are used in infusions for hair, skin, and also for soothing tired eyes. It is a wonderfully useful herb— no wonder Peter Rabbit's mother gave him chamomile tea after his difficult day with Mr. McGregor!

Dill – This herb is familiar for its many culinary uses. In this book I use the seeds for breath freshening.

Fennel Seed – A very aromatic herb with a licorice-like taste. The taste of these seeds are familiar to anyone who has eaten Italian Sausage. An infusion of the seeds makes an aromatic fluid that is good for cleansing facials and reportedly is good for wrinkles. They are also good for breath freshening.

Ground Cinnamon – A familiar smell in baked goods. Used in mouthwash preparations for breath freshening.

Ground Cloves – A lovely seasonal smell in homes all over the country. Also used in mouthwash preparations.

Hops – A herb used in the brewing of beer, but useful to all in a sleep pillow.

Lady's Mantle – The rounded fluted leaves make this a striking plant. Use them in facial washes and masks.

Lavender – An old fashioned scented herb that is making an aromatic comeback. It is used for creams and cleansers. It has the reputation of stimulating and cleansing the skin.

Lemon Balm – A lovely lemony smelling herb that will remind you of the lemon scent in furniture polish preparations. Good for skin cleansing, especially oily skin.

Lemon Verbena – This of all the lemon scented herbs available is the most lemony! Used in sleep pillows.

Mint – A herb that has many different varieties with a distinctive flavor and scent to each one. It is used in baths and facial washes.

Parsley – The green garnish found on your dinner plate can also be used as a breath freshener.

Peppermint – A prolific herb of the mint family used in facial care and baths.

Rosemary – A lovely herb with a fragrance that is somewhat piney used in hair and skin care.

Sage – A herb that is familiar to all cooks is useful in hair and skin care as well.

Thyme – A familiar culinary herb that has a nice aroma. It also has antiseptic and deodorizing properties. Used in deodorants, sleep pillows, and facial scrubs.

Yarrow – A herb found both wild and cultivated. It has astringent properties and is used in skin cleansers.

∞ ESSENTIAL OILS ∞

*C*ssential oils are substances derived from various parts of herbs. These parts could be bark, leaves, flowers, roots, seeds, or fruit depending upon the plant. For example, the essential oils of orange, pettitgraine, and neroli all come from various parts of the orange tree. Orange essential oil comes from the fruit's rind, pettitgraine comes from the leaves and twigs, and neroli comes from the orange blossoms.

Essential oils are very, very concentrated. They are *only* measured by the drop. Their use is primarily through inhalation of the aroma and absorption of the essence through the skin. Essential oils should not be taken internally unless under the direction of a trained aromatherapist, who is a person well educated in the use of essential oils.

It takes different amounts of plant material to make any specific essential oil. For example, it takes sixty thousand rose petals to produce one ounce of pure essential oil of rose, therefore rose essential oil is very pricey. In contrast, it takes 220 pounds of lavender to make 7 pounds of essential oil, so the oil will not be as costly. Do not be dismayed at essential oil prices because there are 120 drops in ⅛ ounce of any essential oil. That is enough essential oil for many, many recipes. If you are limited by the cost of some of the essential oils, check around at herb or natural foods stores. Some of them will sell the more expensive oils by the drop.

If stored in a dark glass container away from heat and light the shelf life is about 2 years. It can be used as a fragrance oil after that but do not expect the therapeutic properties to be intact any longer. Essential oil should not feel "oily" nor should it feel cool like rubbing alcohol—that means it has probably been adulterated. When put in water it should not leave a milky color. This is also a sign that it was adulterated in some way.

Please remember in all recipes in this book to use essential oils instead of fragrance oils. Essential oils have the reputation of doing beneficial things for your skin. Fragrance oils will make you smell good but will not provide the cosmetic benefits of the essential oils. They will likely have synthetic substances in them that can cause sensitivity reactions in some people. I will include in this section a list of essential oils used in my recipes with a brief explanation of their properties. For more information it is a good idea to obtain a detailed aromatherapy book to help you experiment with mixing essential oils. I like to use Valerie Worwood's *The Complete Book of Essential Oils and Aromatherapy*, among others. (See bibliography.) Like herbs, the more you read about essential oils, the better informed you will be in the uses for them.

Avoid using essential oils carelessly. Because of their concentrated form, essential oils must be diluted before coming in contact with your skin and must never be used in or around the eye or other sensitive mucous membranes. Be very careful about what oils and how much to use on infants and children. Consult a reliable aromatherapy book. Pregnant women must also be cautious in their use of essential oils. A partial list of essential oils to avoid for pregnant women are: basil, carrot seed, camphor, cedarwood, cinnamon, clary sage, clove, fennel, frankincense, hyssop, juniper, marjoram, myrrh, oregano, pennyroyal, peppermint, rose, rosemary, sage, thyme, and verbena.

Enjoy working with essential oils. Treat them with the respect they deserve, do not overdo it, and enjoy the aroma when working with them. Keep in mind that essential oils are very volatile and should not be added to hot or very warm mixtures because they will evaporate before you are able to enjoy their benefits.

Here is a list of essential oils used in the recipes in this book:

Basil – Cleansing to skin, it is also antiseptic, toning, and has a spicy aroma.

Bergamot – A lovely smelling essential oil that is deodorizing and has astringent properties. Use on normal or oily skin and hair. Avoid exposing skin with bergamot oil on it to sunlight because it can cause a reaction.

Carrot Seed – Good for use all over the body. Use on irritated, dry, chapped, or wrinkled skin. Useful for dry hair. Also can be used on nails.

Cedarwood – Has astringent and soothing properties. Can be used for stimulating skin and is also useful for troubled skin. The aroma seems very masculine to me. It makes a good choice for aftershave lotion.

Chamomile – Good for dry or normal hair; and sensitive, chapped, normal, wrinkled, or irritated skin. It is also good for lips. It has soothing and toning qualities.

Cinnamon – good for irritated skin.

Clary Sage – Do not confuse this with sage oil, which I do not recommend because of the potential of harmful side effects. Clary sage is deodorizing and good for troubled or wrinkled skin. Its use is not recommended if you have had any alcohol intake because it is reported to cause nightmares when the two are mixed.

Clove – A spicy smelling essential oil that is good for softening calloused skin. Can also be used in mouth care. Use only a very small amount as it has the potential to irritate.

Eucalyptus – Good for oily or irritated skin.

Frankincense – It is astringent, revitalizing, and regenerative to the skin. Good for chapped, mature, and oily skin. Also good for dry hair.

Grapefruit – Good for nails. Also deodorizing.

Jasmine – A most luxurious smelling essential oil. It is extremely high priced—I only use it in bath and body oils for special occasions.

Juniper – Has a clean aroma. Good for normal and oily hair. It has cleansing, toning, and astringent properties, and can be used for oily, irritated, or congested skin.

Lavender – An old fashioned aroma. Very versatile and good for all skin types. Can be used all over the body. It is especially useful when used on chapped skin, burns, sunburn, and wrinkles. It has regenerative and toning properties. Also good for dry or oily hair.

Lemon – As good smelling as the fruit from which it is derived! Recommended for all skin types. Good for lip care and all over the body. Can also be used on sunburn or congested or chapped skin. Use on brittle fingernails. Can also be used on normal blond hair or oily hair. Its cleansing properties make it a good addition to soaps and shampoos.

Lime – Refreshingly fragrant, it has mildly astringent properties and I use it in bath salts.

Myrrh – This has many healing properties and is especially good for mouth and gum care. Good for sensitive, chapped, irritated, or wrinkled skin. Also has some astringent properties.

Orange – Lovely fresh smelling aroma, this essential oil is toning. Good for oily, sensitive, mature, wrinkled, or dry skin.

Palmarosa – Derived from a grass found in Central and South America, it has natural antiseptic and bactericidal properties.

Patchouli – Anybody who was around in the '60s will recognize this scent. Then and now you either loved or hated the aroma. I personally am in the "love it" category for patchouli. It is recommended for all skin types and has deodorizing properties. It can also be used on normal hair.

Peppermint – This essential oil smells like Christmas candy. Good for oily, irritated, or congested skin. Also cooling for sunburn. The aroma is awakening, so don't use in a bath at bedtime.

Pine – A wonderful fragrance to help you feel rejuvenated. I use it in bath salts.

Rose – Good for all skin types, it is toning for wrinkles and regenerative to skin. Also good for chapped skin. Can also be used for lip care. Rose essential oil is one of the most expensive essential oils.

Rose Geranium – Good for lip care. Also good for dry hair. Can be used on sensitive, normal, aged, oily, chapped, dry, or wrinkled skin. This essential oil can be used to replace the scent of rose because it is similar but do not use it to replace the other characteristics of rose essential oil.

Rosemary – Use on wrinkled or oily skin, also good for oily and normal hair. Has astringent and toning properties, stimulates circulation, and is regenerative to skin. Also good for hands and nails.

Rosewood – Deodorizing, slightly toning, and revitalizing. Good for wrinkled or normal skin. Also known as *Bois de Rose*. I think this is also a masculine scent. Try it in aftershave.

Sandalwood – An exotic scent, it is healing, regenerative, moisturizing, and soothing. Good for chapped, mature, oily, irritated, or dry skin. Also good in aftershave or toner for men.

Tangerine – A clean smelling essential oil. Good in lip care products.

Tea Tree – This essential oil has been called a medicine chest in a bottle. It has antibacterial and antifungal properties. I like to use it in lip gloss. It is also good for chapped irritated skin.

Thyme – As soon as you smell this essential oil you will recognize it as an ingredient of a popular medicinal-type mouthwash. It has many antiseptic properties, stimulates circulation, is toning, and good for wrinkles. Can be used on troubled skin. Do not use on children.

Ylang-Ylang – The name means flower of flowers. It has a rich scent and emollient qualities. Use on normal, oily, dry, aged, and mature skin.

TAKING CARE
∽ OF YOUR APPEARANCE ∾
NATURALLY

*D*ifferent cosmetics do help to protect and care for your skin, but before you reach for any jars, bottles, or ingredients there are some other things to do to take care of your appearance.

First of all, get a good night's sleep. It is always obvious when you look at a person whether or not they have slept well. Try not to rely on medications for getting to sleep—a good, natural sleep is much better for you. Try a sleep pillow (see upcoming section) to lull you to sleep with fragrance before reaching into the medicine cabinet. Keep your mind free from that list in your head of things to do tomorrow and forget about the conflict at work. If you don't, all of those things will be rerun over and over in your mind when your eyes close. Also avoid products containing caffeine in the evening—it is a stimulant and will interfere with your attempts to go to sleep.

Another important point about sleeping is to use the softest pillow available. An extra soft pillow is kinder to the delicate skin on your face. It avoids the pushing and stretching of the skin that occurs when using a firmer pillow.

Water both inside and out has a big effect on your appearance. Washing too often is bad for your skin, whether it is oily or dry. Too much washing of oily skin can excessively stimulate the oil glands, making oily skin oilier, while frequent washing of dry skin makes it more dry. Washing the face twice a day should be plenty unless you're cleaning out the garage or mowing the lawn on a humid 90 degree summer day, or some other equally sweaty dirty job. Another point about washing is that it's all right to use soap on any type of skin, including dry skin as long as you don't use harsh deodorant soaps. Soap is alkaline and does alter the acid mantle of the skin briefly, but your skin has the ability to readjust itself. Use a milder soap especially if you have dry or sensitive skin. Only use a small amount of soap and rinse every trace of it from your skin, patting, not rubbing it dry.

Taking baths too frequently can also cause excessive dryness of the skin. Baths that are too warm dry your skin and drain your energy. Lukewarm bath water is much better for you.

Another important factor about moisture is the lack of humidity in your house, especially in the fall and winter. A simple table top humidifier will greatly improve the moisture content of the air. Even bowls of water placed near heat registers will add to the humidity. (Add a few drops of essential oil to the water for a pleasing scent.) Dry air will make your skin and mucous membranes feel very tight and uncomfortable.

Facial steams or facial saunas are another way our faces are exposed to water, but I strongly discourage you from using them. This type of procedure puts a concentrated amount of very hot moist air in contact with your skin, and can be damaging. Facial steams should absolutely not be used on faces that are acne prone, that have very dry skin, or those with broken or fragile capillaries. These procedures also can cause steam burns to your skin if the steam is too hot. Instead, use soft cloths soaked in warm water applied to your face if you wish to open your pores for cleansing, then follow with a toner or astringent.

Drinking enough water to keep your skin well hydrated is also very important. You can put creams and moisturizers on your skin day after day, but unless you keep your body well hydrated you will not look your best. Six to eight 8-ounce glasses of water a day is recommended, more if you are very active and perspiring heavily. Water is the ideal drink for hydration, but other fluids may be taken as well. If you think you aren't losing any body fluid because you're sitting at a desk all day, think again. Even breathing in and out causes you to lose moisture and you perspire even if you lead a sedentary life.

Proper diet is also important not just to your skin but to your entire well-being. Eat lots of fresh fruits and vegetables. Keep fat intake to the recommended 30% or lower of your daily intake. Avoid refined carbohydrates—often these have had all of the nutrients and fiber removed to make the product look nice and white, then the nutrients are artificially put back into the product. This makes no sense to me when all of the nutrients and fiber were there in the first place. There are many books and other information available to you concerning a healthy diet. Read them and stay informed.

The sun is a notorious cause of skin problems. It can give you wrinkles, sunburn, and worst of all, skin cancer. Wear sunscreen, wear a hat when outside, and avoid getting a sunburn. For goodness sake, do not use tanning booths! At the absolute best you are giving your skin the opportunity to age prematurely. At the worst you are causing your skin and body irreversible harm. Avoid them!

Get enough exercise. Take a walk, ride a bicycle, play tag with your children! Get outside and do yard work. Clean the house. You know what you need to do. Get out there and do it.

Finally, take care of your inner self. Resolve your inner tensions and deal with your conflicts. Relax and take some time out for yourself. If you are in a turmoil internally and you are not dealing with it, your looks will be affected. Just taking responsibility for your inner and outer self will give you a fine feeling and boost your self-esteem besides making you look better.

All of these things will help you look your best. Not only will you look better, but you will feel better, which is an added bonus. None of these hints will make you beautiful overnight. It takes some effort and time to achieve an appearance of health and well being. Use common sense and consistently work on all aspects of your life and routine that effect your health and appearance. You will ultimately see results that will be pleasing to you both inside and out.

⨏ GETTING STARTED ⨎

*W*hen you are making the body care products in this book, make small batches in case it doesn't turn out the way you want so you will not waste a large quantity of ingredients. Making small batches will also give it less of a chance to spoil. Even with Vitamin E or tincture of benzoin as a preservative in many of these formulas, keep in mind that the shelf life of these products will not be indefinite. To prolong the shelf life, have all utensils for mixing scrupulously clean. Store products in glass containers when possible and keep away from prolonged heat and direct sunlight. Should any product change color, aroma, develop mold, or develop an "off" odor or appearance discard immediately. Any finished products that need refrigeration will be so noted.

Don't be afraid to try these and have fun while you are doing so. There are many wonderful natural ingredients available to you to make cosmetics. After trying the recipes in this book, review the ingredients list and the herb and essential oils lists, and experiment with custom designing your own products. Switch one oil for another, one clay for another, an essential oil for one that is more suitable to your skin, and/or more pleasing to your senses. For a longer shelf life, use Vitamin E or tincture of benzoin when appropriate. Emulsifiers for creams and lotions are lecithin and/or beeswax. All heated products must be whisked until cool to prevent lumpiness. The recipes will not have the same consistency as commercial preparations. Only use a small amount of the finished products because they are concentrated and a little goes a long way.

The possibilities of combinations are endless. Formulate new recipes yourself, if you're feeling adventuresome. If not, stick with the ones I have developed for you. They have all been tried by me, my family, and friends to make sure that they are useful and usable. Use the ones most suited to your skin and hair type. Enjoy!

⬲ DEODORANT ⬱

*U*nderarm odor occurs when by-products in perspiration break down when exposed to air and bacteria is formed. The following preparations contain ingredients with antibacterial and deodorizing properties. Apply these liquids with cotton pads to the underarm area and let dry before putting on clothing.

DEODORANT NO. 1

1 Tbsp. pure grain alcohol
2 drops lemon essential oil
2 drops lavender essential oil
1 drop tea tree essential oil
1 drop thyme essential oil

Mix above ingredients together, then add:

1 Tbsp. witch hazel
10 drops grapefruit seed
    extract

Mix well. Shake before using.

DEODORANT NO. 2

1 Tbsp. rubbing alcohol
2 drops tea tree essential oil
1 drop lemon essential oil
2 drops thyme essential oil

Mix the above ingredients and place in a closed glass container.

Then add:

1 Tbsp. witch hazel
10 drops grapefruit seed
    extract

Shake well before using.

DEODORANT NO. 3

Don't be concerned about the odor of vinegar in this formula. You cannot smell it after it is applied, so you won't have the odor of a pickle!

1 Tbsp. cider vinegar or white
    vinegar
3 drops bergamot essential oil
3 drops patchouli essential oil
15 drops grapefruit seed
    extract
1 Tbsp. witch hazel

Mix above ingredients. Store in a glass container. Shake before using.

DEODORANT NO. 4

2 Tbsp. cider vinegar or white
vinegar
5 drops patchouli essential oil
3 drops lemon essential oil
2 drops myrrh essential oil
10 drops grapefruit seed
extract
2 Tbsp. witch hazel
Mix above ingredients. Store in a
glass container. Shake well before
using.

DEODORANT NO. 5

2 Tbsp. witch hazel
25 drops grapefruit seed
extract
5 drops tincture of benzoin
8 drops lavender essential oil
5 drops tea tree essential oil
Mix above ingredients. Store in a
glass container. Shake well before
using.

DEODORANT NO. 6

2 Tbsp. pure grain alcohol
3 drops peppermint essential
oil
1 drop rosemary essential oil
1 drop juniper essential oil.
Mix above ingredients. Store in a
glass container. Shake well before
using.

DEODORANT NO. 7

2 Tbsp. cider vinegar or white
vinegar
3 drops thyme essential oil
2 drops lemon essential oil
2 drops rosemary essential oil
Mix above ingredients, then add:
1 Tbsp. witch hazel
Mix well. Store in a glass container.
Shake well before using.

DEODORANT NO. 8

2 Tbsp. witch hazel
2 drops myrrh essential oil
2 drops cinnamon essential oil
4 drops lavender essential oil
1 drop thyme essential oil
1 drop juniper essential oil
Mix ingredients well. Store in a
glass container. Shake well before
using.

⨍ EYE CARE ⨍

*Y*our eyes are so very important, and must be treated with the utmost care. It is not unusual for one's eyes to become reddened on occasion from pollutants in the air or from lack of sleep. These problems can easily be taken care of yourself. However, report any redness that doesn't go away and/or unusual drainage or discharge from your eyes to a health care professional. Do not introduce any drops or foreign substances into your eyes without professional supervision.

The skin around the eyes also requires extra care because it is more fragile than the skin on the rest of your face. It should not be rubbed or scrubbed hard, as this will stretch the skin too much and it cannot spring back readily. Avoid any concentrated substances like essential oils around your eyes—they can make your eyes burn and sting, reddening the eyes and making them watery. Also get adequate sleep to assure your eyes are looking their best. Eye care products are made in very small quantities to keep the chance of bacterial growth to a minimum.

There are several substances that are safe and gentle to use around your eyes. Many of them are classics and work very well. For tired, reddened, and/or irritated eyes or for dark circles under your eyes, try some of these remedies.

EYE SOOTHER NO. 1

Take 2 chamomile tea bags and place in hot distilled water. Allow water to cool to lukewarm and remove the tea bags and squeeze out the excess water and place the bags on closed eyes. Rest for 15 minutes with tea bags in place. Remove from eyes. (You could save the chamomile infusion and store in the refrigerator for use as a hair rinse or as a facial rinse. Use in 2 to 3 days.)

EYE SOOTHER NO. 2

2 Tbsp. dried calendula
   blossoms
⅓ cup distilled water

Simmer the blossoms in the water for 15 minutes. Strain and allow the infusion to cool. Soak gauze squares, clean cloth squares, or cotton pads in the infusion, squeeze out excess, and place on closed eyes. Rest for 15 minutes, then remove.

EYE SOOTHER NO. 3

3 Tbsp. crushed fennel seeds
⅓ cup distilled water

Simmer the seeds in water for 15 minutes. Strain the infusion and let cool. Soak gauze squares, clean cloth squares, or cotton pads in infusion, squeeze out excess and place on closed eyes for 15 minutes.

AROUND THE EYE OIL

Avoid rich creams and oils around the eye—they can promote puffiness and even possible allergic reactions, causing the eyes to not only be puffy but reddened! This formula is very light. Use sparingly.

⅛ tsp. rosehip seed oil
10 drops evening primrose oil
10 drops Vitamin E—use 400
   IU per gelcap or
   concentrated liquid (32,000
   IU per fluid ounce) form
10 drops jojoba oil

Mix ingredients. Use just a drop or two and gently massage into the skin around your eyes.

∽ LIP CARE ∾

CITRUS LIP GLOSS

When I sent a sample of this for my friend to try, she called to say, "This tastes good, send me more!" The citrus essential oils and honey combine to make this gloss a tasty product that will keep your lips soft and moist for some time.

   3 Tbsp. sweet almond oil
   2 tsp. beeswax (pearls or solid
      beeswax grated and
      measured)
   1 tsp. aloe vera gel
   1 tsp. honey
   800 IU Vitamin E
   4 drops lemon essential oil
   3 drops tangerine essential oil

Melt beeswax and almond oil together in a heatproof container over boiling water. When melted, remove from heat. Add honey and Vitamin E, mixing briskly with a wire whisk. Add aloe vera gel, and continue to mix briskly. When almost cool and set, add the essential oils and mix. Do not stop whisking while the mixture is cooling—the ingredients could separate and you would have a lumpy product. Store in a low widemouthed jar.

LIP GLOSS

This is a more "serious" lip gloss for protection and moisturizing with the coconut oil and carrot seed essential oil. It also includes the healing properties of tea tree essential oil. Not as tasty as the first formula, but is excellent in its protective and emollient qualities.

3 Tbsp. apricot kernel oil
2 tsp. beeswax (pearls or solid beeswax grated and measured)
1 tsp. coconut oil
800 IU Vitamin E
5 drops carrot seed essential oil
3 drops lemon essential oil
2 drops tea tree essential oil

Melt beeswax, apricot kernel oil, and coconut oil over boiling water in a heat proof container. When melted, remove from heat. Add Vitamin E, mixing with wire whisk. Just before mixture is set add all three essential oils and mix well. Do not stop whisking while product is cooling or it will get lumpy. Store in a low widemouthed glass or plastic jar.

EXTRA CARE FOR LIPS

This recipe is very protective, tastes good, and has a good consistency.

3 tsp. beeswax (pearls or solid beeswax grated and measured)
3 tsp. avocado oil
1 tsp. vegetable glycerine
½ tsp. honey
⅛ tsp. lecithin
800 IU Vitamin E
4 drops tea tree essential oil
6 drops grapefruit essential oil

Melt beeswax and avocado oil over boiling water in a heatproof container. When melted, remove from heat. Mix honey and vegetable glycerine separately. Add Vitamin E and lecithin to the beeswax and oil mixture. Slowly add the honey and vegetable glycerine mixture. This will set up very quickly. Add essential oils and mix well. Store in a low widemouthed glass or plastic jar.

☙ MOUTH AND TOOTH CARE ☙

*T*here are several natural alternatives to commercial toothpaste preparations. My recipes include the classic tooth cleaning ingredients baking soda and/or salt. (Use regular table salt for the salt used in these recipes.) Mouth freshening preparations are as close as your herb bed or spice cabinet. Also, try this simple mechanical way to freshen your mouth—brush your tongue when you brush your teeth—it really helps to decrease mouth odor.

TOOTH CLEANER NO. 1

This preparation has a medicinal but not unpleasant taste, and your mouth will feel very fresh when you are finished.

   1 tsp. baking soda
   1 drop thyme essential oil
Mix and put on dampened toothbrush to use.

TOOTH CLEANER NO. 2

Fresh and pleasant tasting!

   ¼ tsp. table salt
   ¼ tsp. baking soda
   1 drop clove essential oil
   1 drop peppermint essential oil
Mix and put on dampened toothbrush to use.

TOOTH CLEANER NO. 3

Myrrh is a tried and true herb for the mouth and gums. This preparation has a very invigorating feel in the mouth.

   1 tsp. table salt
   1 tsp. baking soda
   2 drops myrrh essential oil
Mix ingredients, and put on dampened toothbrush to use.

TOOTH CLEANER NO. 4

   ½ tsp. baking soda
   ½ tsp. table salt
   1 drop clove essential oil
Mix ingredients, and put on dampened toothbrush to use.

TOOTH CLEANER NO. 5

Clay helps to remove mouth odor.
¼ tsp. baking soda
⅛ tsp. fuller's earth
1 drop myrrh essential oil
Mix ingredients, and put on dampened toothbrush to use.

MOUTHWASH NO. 1

This mouthwash does not have a sweet taste like commercial preparations because it does not contain any artificial sweeteners.
1 Tbsp. pure grain alcohol
1 drop *each* clove essential oil,
    cinnamon essential oil,
    myrrh essential oil, and tea
    tree essential oil
¾ cup distilled water
Add essential oils to the alcohol and shake well, then add distilled water. This will be a milky looking fluid. Store in a capped bottle.

MOUTHWASH NO. 2

1 Tbsp. pure grain alcohol
1 drop myrrh essential oil
1 drop peppermint essential
    oil
½ cup distilled water
Add essential oils to alcohol in a closed container. Shake well, then add distilled water. Solution will turn a milky color.

MOUTHWASH NO. 3

This mouthwash is very spicy.
½ tsp. ground cloves
½ tsp. ground cinnamon
½ tsp. fennel seed
2 Tbsp. pure grain alcohol
1 cup distilled water
Add spices to alcohol. Cover and store in a glass container for 3 days. Strain through paper coffee filter. Add the distilled water. Mixture will be a cloudy brown color. Bottle in a glass container.

MOUTH FRESHENER NO. 1

Chew a sprig of fresh parsley—this really does work. Now you know why restaurants use this on your plate—and you thought it was just for garnish!

MOUTH FRESHENER NO. 2

Chew ½ tsp. fennel seeds. This has a strong licorice-like flavor.

⌒ HAND CLEANSERS ⌒

Some of these recipes are as easy as reaching into the pantry or refrigerator. As with all recipes in this book, ingredients can be substituted according to your needs and preferences.

HEAVY DUTY CLEANER

My husband used this after working out in the garage most of one afternoon and found that it worked quite well.

Rub about a teaspoon of full strength wheat germ oil onto grimy hands, then wipe off with a damp towel. This will cleanse your hands plus leave them feeling soft.

CITRUS CLEANER

What could be simpler? Especially nice to eliminate food smells from your hands when preparing a meal.

Cut 1 fresh lemon in half. Take the cut side of the lemon and rub the pulp onto your hands, squeezing the lemon a bit to extract some of the juice. Rub your hands together with the juice then rinse off with water. Wipe hands dry.

PICNIC CLEANSERS

When we cook out I like to put a bowl of this on the table with paper towels to dip into it for cleanup while everyone is outside. It takes care of hands smeared with barbecue sauce and eliminates unnecessary trips into the house.

  1 bowl of water
  2–3 drops of lemon, lime,
     orange, or tangerine
     essential oil, your choice.
Add essential oil to the bowl of water. Place the bowl on your picnic table with paper towels next to it.

WATERLESS HAND CLEANER

The lemon essential oil in this recipe gives this product a clean fresh smell and the castor oil helps to keep hands soft.

1 Tbsp. fuller's earth
½ tsp. liquid dish detergent
2 Tbsp. castor oil
¼ tsp. tincture of benzoin
3 drops lemon essential oil

Mix together and place in a wide mouth jar. Rub about 1 teaspoonful into dirty hands, then wipe off with a damp paper towel or damp cloth.

CREAMY SOAP IN A JAR

Not just for hands—try it in the bath, too.

½ cup grated pure or castile
   soap
1 cup distilled water
pinch borax
1 Tbsp. witch hazel
1 Tbsp. sweet almond oil
3 drops lavender essential oil

Heat water in a saucepan—add borax to water and dissolve. Add soap to water and boil until soap is dissolved. Remove from heat-whisk in witch hazel and sweet almond oil. Allow to cool slightly, then add essential oil. The more you whisk the preparation, the fluffier it becomes. Store in a low widemouthed jar.

HANDWASHING SOAP

This is a good kitchen hand soap. It has a lovely consistency and could even be used in the bath.

½ cup distilled water
scant ¼ cup witch hazel
¼ cup grated pure soap
¾ tsp. arrowroot powder
15 drops grapefruit seed
   extract
5 drops lemon essential oil

Boil water. Add soap to dissolve on low heat. Add arrowroot powder after soap is dissolved and whisk until it too is dissolved. Cook over low heat for about 15 minutes, continuing to whisk. Remove from heat. Add witch hazel and stir. Allow to cool for several minutes, then add grapefruit seed extract and lemon essential oil and stir. Stir occasionally while cooling so ingredients remain mixed together. Store in a low widemouthed jar.

HAND CREAMS

*A*s a housewife and serious gardener, I find that my hands take a lot of abuse. When I was working on these recipes I was especially trying to obtain products that are protective, softening, and healing when needed. I think you will find that these products meet all of these needs. All of these preparations can be used on the body as well as the hands. If you do not like a preparation's consistency, adjust it as follows: If it is too thick, add more oil in 1 tsp. increments. If it is too thin, add more beeswax in ½ tsp. increments. In rare instances oil will separate out of some of these recipes. Simply stir it back in before using.

CREAMY HONEY

This preparation is a rich golden color with lots of healthy ingredients for your skin.

  1 Tbsp. beeswax (pearls or
     solid beeswax grated and
     measured)
  1 Tbsp. shea butter
  1 Tbsp. wheat germ oil
  1 Tbsp. honey
  ½ tsp. rosehip seed oil
  800 IU Vitamin E
  2 drops lemon essential oil
  2 drops sandalwood essential
     oil
  2 drops rose geranium
     essential oil

Melt beeswax, shea butter, and wheat germ oil in a heatproof container over boiling water. Remove from heat when melted. Whisk in honey, rosehip seed oil, and Vitamin E. Continue to whisk as mixture cools. When mixture is almost set, add essential oils and mix well. Store in a low widemouthed jar.

AVOCADO HAND CREAM

Avocado oil is very rich and makes your skin feel so soft. That is why I made it the primary ingredient for this cream. Try it and see what you think.

1 tsp. beeswax (pearls or solid beeswax grated and measured)
1 Tbsp. avocado oil
1 tsp. jojoba oil
20 drops evening primrose oil
800 IU Vitamin E
3 drops patchouli essential oil
5 drops carrot seed essential oil
2 drops frankincense essential oil
3 drops rosewood essential oil

Melt beeswax and avocado oil in a heatproof container over boiling water. Remove from heat when melted. Add evening primrose oil, jojoba oil, and Vitamin E to the mixture and whisk until blended. Whisk the mixture frequently as it is cooling. When mixture is almost set, add essential oils, mixing well. Store in a widemouthed jar.

SOFTEN YOUR HANDS CREAM

I gave some of this cream to my 89 year old friend to try—she loved the aroma and consistency.

1 tsp. coconut oil
½ tsp. wheat germ oil
1 Tbsp. shea butter
½ tsp. vegetable glycerine
15 drops grapefruit seed extract
400 IU Vitamin E
6 drops lavender essential oil
6 drops rose geranium essential oil

Melt coconut oil, wheat germ oil, and shea butter over boiling water. Mix glycerine and grapefruit seed extract separately and set aside. When oil mixture is melted, remove from heat. Whisk in Vitamin E and the glycerine mixture. When preparation is cooling and almost set, add essential oils and mix well. Keep in mind that shea butter preparations take longer to set—be patient. Store in low widemouthed container.

MY OWN HAND CREAM

"What makes this so smooth?" asked my mother. The secret is the shea butter, which gives any preparation a lovely creamy consistency. She uses it all over her body with very satisfactory results.

2 Tbsp. shea butter
1 Tbsp. apricot kernel oil
1 tsp. avocado oil
½ tsp. rosehip seed oil
½ tsp. rosewater
800 IU Vitamin E
6 drops lavender essential oil

Melt shea butter, apricot kernel oil, and avocado oil over boiling water. When melted, remove from heat. Add rosehip seed oil and Vitamin E and whisk. When mixture is setting up and almost cool, add rosewater and the essential oil. It takes melted preparations with shea butter more time to solidify, so be patient. Store in a widemouthed jar.

HEALING HAND CREAM

So thick it is almost a salve, this is a heavy duty cream with many soothing ingredients. Use sparingly whenever you need extra care for your hands.

  2 tsp. beeswax (pearls or solid
      beeswax grated and
      measured)
  2 Tbsp. castor oil
  1 Tbsp. wheat germ oil
  10 drops jojoba oil
  ½ tsp. lecithin
  15 drops grapefruit seed
      extract
  800 IU Vitamin E
  3 drops chamomile essential oil
  4 drops myrrh essential oil
  4 drops tea tree essential oil

Melt beeswax, castor oil, and wheat germ oil over boiling water. When melted, remove from heat and add jojoba oil and Vitamin E. Whisk together. Add lecithin and grapefruit seed extract. Continue whisking. When almost set, add essential oils and mix well. Store in a widemouthed jar.

RICHLY SCENTED HAND CREAM

You will truly feel pampered when using this richly scented cream. One of my friends used it on her face with no problems, and she has dry very sensitive skin.

  2 Tbsp. shea butter
  1 Tbsp. avocado oil
  1 tsp. rosehip seed oil
  1 tsp. lecithin
  1 Tbsp. rosewater
  800 IU Vitamin E
  5 drops ylang-ylang essential
      oil
  2 drops patchouli essential oil
  4 drops lemon essential oil

Melt shea butter and avocado oil over boiling water. Remove from heat when mixture is melted. Add rosehip seed oil, Vitamin E, and lecithin. Whisk together. Add rosewater and whisk into oil mixture. Allow preparation to cool and when it is almost set, add all essential oils and mix. Store in a low widemouthed jar.

"NOT JUST FOR BABY" CREAM

I made this for a friend's baby. It is very protective and soothing. All of the ingredients are safe to use as a diaper cream or all over the infant's skin if needed. Don't forget, you can use it too!

2 Tbsp. beeswax (pearls or solid beeswax grated and measured)

3½ Tbsp. castor oil

1 Tbsp. sweet almond oil

10 drops jojoba oil

800 IU Vitamin E

1 drop chamomile essential oil

1 drop lavender essential oil

Melt beeswax and oils except for jojoba oil over boiling water. When melted, remove from heat. Add jojoba oil and Vitamin E and whisk. When almost cool and set, add essential oils and mix thoroughly. Store in a low wide-mouthed jar.

COLD CREAM

I used chamomile for its soothing qualities, but you could change that to another essential oil if you preferred. One of my friends uses this on her face while showering, lets it soak in throughout the shower, then takes it off. She says it "keeps my winter skin soft and moist."

3 Tbsp. pure olive oil

1 Tbsp. aloe vera gel

1 Tbsp. shea butter

2 tsp. beeswax (pearls or solid beeswax grated and measured)

1 Tbsp. rosewater

¼ tsp. lecithin

800 IU Vitamin E

3 drops chamomile essential oil

Melt olive oil, shea butter, and beeswax together in a heatproof container over boiling water. Remove from heat when melted. Add Vitamin E and lecithin and mix well. Separately mix rosewater and aloe vera gel together. Slowly combine the two mixtures. Continue stirring with the whisk. When the preparation is cooled, add the essential oil. Store in a low widemouthed jar.

LIGHT CREAM

The calendula infused oil adds a therapeutic touch. A friend had surgery and came home with "sheet burns" on her elbows. She used this cream to help heal them with good results.

2 tsp. beeswax (pearls or solid beeswax grated and measured)

3 tsp. coconut oil

2 tsp. calendula infused oil (See instructions for making in the bath and body oil section)

2 tsp. vegetable glycerine

3 tsp. rosewater

800 IU Vitamin E

¼ tsp. lecithin

10 drops carrot seed essential oil

5 drops rosewood essential oil

2 drops frankincense essential oil

Melt beeswax, coconut oil, and calendula oil together over boiling water. When melted, remove from heat. Add lecithin and Vitamin E to the oil mixture and mix well. Combine glycerine and rosewater together separately. Slowly add rosewater and glycerine mixture to oil mixture, mixing continually. When the mixture is cool and almost set, add all essential oils and mix well. Store in a low widemouthed jar.

APRICOT HAND CREAM

1 Tbsp. apricot kernel oil
1½ Tbsp. coconut oil
2 tsp. beeswax (pearls or solid beeswax grated and measured)
1½ Tbsp. vegetable glycerine
800 IU Vitamin E
3 drops bergamot essential oil

Melt beeswax and oils in a heatproof container over boiling water. When melted, remove from heat. Add Vitamin E to the oil mixture. Whisk in the glycerine a little at a time. Continue whisking until preparation is well mixed and almost set, then stir in essential oil. Store in a low widemouthed jar.

MOISTURIZER

2 tsp. beeswax (pearls or solid beeswax grated and measured)
1 Tbsp. sweet almond oil

1 tsp. avocado oil
1 tsp. apricot kernel oil
1 Tbsp. coconut oil
1 Tbsp. vegetable glycerine
1 Tbsp. rosewater
1 Tbsp. aloe vera gel
¼ tsp. lecithin
800 IU Vitamin E
6 drops lemon essential oil

Melt beeswax and oils over boiling water. When melted, remove from heat. Add lecithin and Vitamin E to mixture. Separately mix glycerine, rosewater, and aloe vera gel together. Slowly add the rosewater mixture to the oil mixture, whisking continuously. When the preparation is almost cool, add the essential oil and mix well. Store in a low widemouthed jar.

"BUTTERY" RICH BODY BALM

The richness of shea butter and cocoa butter are combined in this recipe to make a lovely cream for all over your body.

1 Tbsp. shea butter
2 tsp. cocoa butter
2 tsp. apricot kernel oil
800 IU Vitamin E
1 tsp. aloe vera gel
¼ tsp. lecithin
5 drops grapefruit seed extract
3 drops lemon essential oil

3 drops rose geranium
essential oil

Melt the butters and oil together over boiling water. Remove from heat when melted. Add Vitamin E and lecithin. Whisk in aloe vera gel and grapefruit seed extract. When almost cool add essential oils. Mix well. Store in a widemouthed jar.

MY FAVORITE INGREDIENTS FORMULA

2 Tbsp. shea butter
1 Tbsp. avocado oil
½ tsp. beeswax (pearls or solid grated and measured)
1 Tbsp. rosewater
¼ tsp. lecithin
10 drops grapefruit seed extract
800 IU Vitamin E
5 drops carrot seed essential oil
3 drops chamomile essential oil
4 drops lavender essential oil
2 drops lemon essential oil

Melt butter, beeswax, and oil in a heatproof container over boiling water. Remove from heat when melted. Mix grapefruit seed extract and rosewater together. Add Vitamin E and lecithin to the oil mixture. Slowly add the rosewater mixture to the oil mixture, whisking continuously. When the cream is almost set and cool, add the essential oils. Store in a low widemouthed jar.

DAILY HAND CARE CREAM

Thick, rich, and easily absorbed.

2 tsp. beeswax (pearls or solid grated and measured)
3 tsp. shea butter
1 tsp. cocoa butter
2 tsp. avocado oil
2 tsp. vegetable glycerine
¼ tsp. lecithin
800 IU Vitamin E
2 drops chamomile essential oil
2 drops lavender essential oil
1 drop rosemary essential oil

Melt the beeswax, butter, and oil together over boiling water. Remove from heat when they are melted. Add Vitamin E and lecithin to the mixture. Slowly add the glycerine, mixing with a whisk as you pour it. When mixture is almost set and cool, add the essential oils. Store in a widemouthed jar.

CALENDULA CREAM

The healing properties of calendula in the infused oil makes this an appropriate choice for troubled hardworking skin.

1 Tbsp. calendula infused oil (See instructions for making in the bath and body oil section of this book.)
1 Tbsp. avocado oil

1 tsp. beeswax (pearls or solid beeswax grated and measured)

1 Tbsp. coconut oil

20 drops jojoba oil

5 drops carrot seed essential oil

5 drops lemon essential oil

3 drops rosemary essential oil

800 IU Vitamin E

Melt the beeswax and all the oils except for jojoba oil over boiling water. When melted remove from heat. Whisk the Vitamin E and jojoba oil into the mixture. When almost cool and set, whisk in all essential oils. Store in a low widemouthed jar.

PROTECTIVE LOTION

This liquid preparation is good to put on your hands before you expose them to cold wet conditions. The lanolin serves as a barrier and the cocoa butter is moisturizing.

2 tsp. castor oil

1 tsp. lanolin

1½ tsp. cocoa butter

800 IU Vitamin E

5 drops lavender essential oil

3 drops tea tree essential oil

Melt the castor oil, lanolin, and cocoa butter over boiling water. When melted, remove from heat. Whisk the Vitamin E into the mixture. When cool add the essential oils, mixing well. Store in a bottle or jar.

HERBAL CREAM

2 tsp. calendula infused oil

1 tsp. chamomile infused oil (See instructions for making both infused oils in the body and bath oil section of this book.)

1 tsp. castor oil

2 tsp. beeswax grated and measured or pearls

¼ tsp. lecithin

800 IU Vitamin E

1 tsp. aloe vera gel

5 drops carrot seed essential oil

4 drops orange essential oil

2 drops rosemary essential oil

2 drops rosewood essential oil

In a heatproof glass bowl over boiling water, melt the oils and the beeswax. Remove from heat and add the Vitamin E and lecithin and mix well. Add the aloe vera gel and mix using a whisk. When mixture has cooled and is almost set, add all of the essential oils. Store in a low widemouthed glass container.

∾ SLEEP PILLOWS ∾

If you have trouble sleeping, try one of these pillows. Resting your head on the wonderful aromas will help lull you to sleep. These are not full size pillows. They are made to tuck between your pillow and pillow case so that it is anchored to stay under your head. They can also be "fancied up" in various fabrics and laces for gift giving, or just to treat yourself if you wish.

I have used cellulose chips as a fixative for the essential oils in these recipes. Many recipes for sleep pillows call for orris root as a fixative agent, but orris root is a substance that many people, myself included, are allergic to. In susceptible people it can cause very severe headaches, so I personally never use it.

SLEEP PILLOW

Hops is typically used in brewing beer, but it is the primary ingredient in sleep pillows because it is reported to contain a substance that induces sleep.

½ cup dried hops
¼ cup dried lemon verbena
¼ cup dried lavender
   blossoms
2 Tbsp. cellulose chips
4 drops lemon essential oil
4 drops lavender essential oil

Mix the essential oils into cellulose chips in a glass bowl. Cover and let sit for four hours or more. The longer you let these two ingredients blend, the better the aroma from the essential oils will be. Mix in the dried herbs. Make two little fabric envelopes 6 inches square. Divide the mixture into two parts and place in fabric envelopes and sew shut.

LAVENDER SLEEP PILLOW

The lavender and bergamot are so fragrant in this recipe.

    1 cup dried hops
    1 cup dried lavender blossoms
    ¼ cup dried thyme
    3 Tbsp. cellulose chips
    10 drops lavender essential oil
    10 drops bergamot essential
       oil

Add essential oils to cellulose chips. Mix well and place in a glass bowl. Cover and let sit overnight to allow oils to absorb into cellulose. Mix in the dried herbs the next day. Place in 2–6 inch square pillows.

SWEET DREAMS SLEEP PILLOW

This pillow has a very sweet smell thanks to the chamomile blossoms and the essential oils

    1 cup dried hops
    ½ cup dried chamomile
       blossoms
    2 Tbsp. cellulose chips
    2 drops rose geranium
       essential oil
    2 drops ylang-ylang essential
       oil

Mix the essential oils into the cellulose chips in a glass bowl. Cover and let sit overnight, then mix with herbs. Make a 6 inch square fabric pillow, place mixture into it, and sew shut.

AROMATIC SLEEP PILLOW

The catnip and rosemary essential oil help to make this sleep pillow a good one if you have a cold.

    ¼ cup dried hops
    ¼ cup dried catnip
    ¼ cup dried lemon balm
    ¼ cup cellulose chips
    2 Tbsp. dried lavender
       blossoms
    6 drops rosemary essential oil
    3 drops lavender essential oil

Add essential oils to cellulose chips in a glass bowl. Cover and let sit overnight. Mix with dried herbs and place mixture into a 6 inch square fabric envelope and sew shut.

❦ BODY POWDER ❦

𝓘 have tried many body powder recipes from different magazines and books, and most of them produce a clumpy mess that won't easily shake from a container. The secret to a smooth powder that shakes easily from a container is the addition of clay. This not only improves the texture of the powder but also adds to its absorbency.

Most commercial preparations contain talc which is a potential lung irritant. Avoid exposure to products containing talc when possible.

I always use a shaker container of some type to dispense the powders I make. Using powder puffs over and over bothers me for aesthetic and hygienic reasons.

BODY POWDER

This is a luxurious smelling powder. The fragrance may be too rich for some but the essentials oils could be adjusted to your needs and liking. The powder itself can keep you feeling fresh all day!

1 Tbsp. arrowroot powder
1 Tbsp. kaolin
1 Tbsp. baking soda
3 drops rose geranium
   essential oil
2 drops jasmine essential oil

Mix the arrowroot powder, clay, and baking soda together. Add the essential oils and mix well. Let sit in a glass container covered for several hours for the oils to absorb into the mixture. Put in a shaker container. Any leftover powder should be stored in a glass jar with a tight lid.

SWEET-SMELLING POWDER

1 cup arrowroot powder
¼ cup baking soda
¼ cup clay (fuller's earth,
   kaolin, or green clay, your
   choice.)
7 drops lavender essential oil
7 drops orange essential oil
2 drops lemon essential oil

Mix arrowroot powder, clay, and baking soda thoroughly. Add essential oils and mix well. Let sit covered in a glass container for several hours. Place in shaker container. Store any leftover powder in a glass container with a tight lid.

CHAMOMILE POWDER

So soothing with the chamomile flowers and essential oil included.

1 cup arrowroot powder
¼ cup kaolin
¼ cup baking soda
1 Tbsp. ground and sifted
   dried chamomile blossoms
8 drops orange essential oil
4 drops chamomile essential
   oil

Add all ingredients together and mix well. Let sit covered in a glass container for several days before using. Put in shaker container for use. Store any leftover powder in a glass container with a tight lid.

Variation: Substitute ground sifted dried lavender blossoms and lavender essential oil for the chamomile blossoms and chamomile essential oil.

∽ BATH TIME ∽

*E*veryone has seen the pictures of people luxuriating in a bathtub filled to the brim with foamy suds and candles lit all around. This is not something many of us get to do very often, but 15 minutes of our time isn't impossible to set aside for a good soak to soothe our nerves and soften our skin. Try to take time out for this activity occasionally. You'll be glad you did. Keep bathwater pleasantly warm—if it is too hot it will be a drain on your energy.

BATH BAG HERBS

Sew up a little 2" by 3" muslin pouch with a little drawstring to hold these herbs. It can be rinsed and used over and over again.

   1 Tbsp. dried lavender
      blossoms
   1 Tbsp. dried rosemary
   1 Tbsp. dried mint
   1 Tbsp. dried chamomile
      blossoms

Mix dried herbs and place in bath bag, closing tightly. Put bag in 1 quart boiling water and simmer for 10 minutes. Turn off heat and let bag sit in water until cool. Add the infusion and bag to a tub of running warm water. Soak in the tub and inhale the aroma, using the bag of herbs as a washcloth.

SOOTHING BATH

Oatmeal is very soothing to all skin types, but especially good if you suffer from dry itchy skin.

   2 Tbsp. oatmeal
   5 drops essential oil, your
      choice

Put essential oil into oatmeal and mix well. Place mixture into a bath bag. Tie bag to the water faucet of your tub while the water is running. Use bag as a washcloth.

SUMMER BATH

Good anytime of year, but an especially "cooling" mix of herbs for summer use. It is also good for softening skin.

    1 Tbsp. dried mint
    1 Tbsp. dried ground lemon
      peel
    2 Tbsp. dried milk powder

Place ingredients in bath bag. Tie bath bag under the faucet of your bathtub while the water is running. Use bag as a washcloth.

WAKE UP BATH

The grapefruit/lavender/mint mixture has a very awakening effect.

    2 Tbsp. ground oatmeal
    1 Tbsp. dried lavender
      blossoms
    5 drops grapefruit essential oil
    2 drops peppermint essential
      oil

Add essential oil to oatmeal. Mix lavender blossoms with oatmeal mixture. Place in bath bag. Tie under the faucet of your tub while the water is running. Use bag as a washcloth.

INVIGORATING BATH SALTS

Use these after being on the go all day to rejuvenate you for an evening's worth of work or play. Sea salt is supposed to draw impurities from your body. The aroma of this recipe may seem a bit strong to you, but when the salts are diluted in your bath water it will be quite pleasant. This would make a great gift. Put in a pretty glass jar with a scoop tied to it.

    1 cup sea salt
    8 drops lime essential oil
    6 drops eucalyptus essential
      oil
    3 drops pine essential oil
    4 drops peppermint essential
      oil
    5 drops lavender essential oil

Put salt in a glass container and add essential oils, stirring after each addition. Cover and let sit for 2 hours, then stir again. Cover and let sit for 2 more hours and stir again. Use ¼ cup at a time in bath water for a good soak. Pour mixture directly under faucet to help the crystals dissolve.

Variations: Try other essential oils according to your needs and/ or preferences. Do not exceed the 26 drops of essential oil to 1 cup of sea salt.

MILK BATH

This is a legendary bath used by some of history's famous beauties. Milk has a softening effect on the skin.

    1 cup dried milk powder
    5–6 drops essential oil, your
      choice

Add essential oil to milk. Add to bath water for a fragrant soak.

WATER SOFTENING BATH

    ½ cup borax
    10 drops essential oil, your
      choice

Mix the borax and 5 drops of essential oil together. Store in a closed glass container. The next day, add 5 more drops of essential oil. Stir and close container. Use 2 Tbsp. mixture in each bath.

∽ SOAPS ∽

I have always loved the idea of making custom designed soaps with natural ingredients, but when I have picked up recipes to make them I become intimidated by the quantity of ingredients involved and the strong lye that has to be handled. Finally, I have come across a quicker, less hazardous way of making soap with herbs and/or essential oils added as I wish. The types of bar soaps used in these recipes are castile soap or pure white soap with no added fragrance. Both of these kinds of soap lather well. When forming the mixtures into balls, wet your hands with water or rosewater so that the mixture will not stick to your hands and so that the soap balls have a shiny finished look to them.

OATMEAL-LAVENDER SOAP

1 4-ounce bar of pure soap, grated
2 Tbsp. distilled water
1 Tbsp. apricot kernel oil
2 Tbsp. ground lavender blossoms
2 tsp. ground oatmeal
3 drops chamomile essential oil
3 drops peppermint essential oil

Mix soap, water, and oil, and let sit for at least one hour. Add ground lavender blossoms and oatmeal. Mix well. Put mixture into a blender or food processor. Add essential oils one drop at a time, mixing well after each addition. Remove mixture and wet hands to form soap into balls. Place on waxed paper to dry and harden. After soap balls are dry, wrap in plastic wrap or waxed paper to store.

GARDENER'S SOAP

The cornmeal helps to clean grubby soiled hands.

> 1 4-ounce bar of pure soap, grated
> 1 Tbsp. cornmeal
> 2 Tbsp. wheat germ oil
> 1 tsp. coconut oil
> 5 drops palmarosa essential oil

Melt soap and oils in a pan over very low heat until the mixture is mushy and workable. Remove from heat. Add the essential oil and cornmeal and mix well. Form into balls and place on waxed paper to harden. Wrap each soap ball in waxed paper or plastic wrap to store.

LEMON CALENDULA SOAP

Refreshing aroma and healing qualities combined into one soap—a useful and enjoyable combination!

> 1 4-ounce bar castile soap, grated
> 2 Tbsp. rosewater
> 1 Tbsp. calendula infused oil (See recipe in the bath and body oil section of this book.)
> 5 drops lemon essential oil

Mix soap, rosewater, and oil in a glass bowl. Cover and let sit overnight. Place mixture in a food processor or a blender and mix thoroughly. Add essential oil one drop at a time mixing thoroughly after each addition. Form mixture into balls and let sit on waxed paper to harden. Wrap each soap ball in waxed paper or plastic wrap to store.

ALOE SOAP

A clean smelling soap that is one of my favorites.

> 1 4-ounce bar castile soap, grated
> 2 Tbsp. aloe vera gel
> 1½ Tbsp. rosewater
> 30 drops evening primrose oil
> 6 drops tangerine essential oil
> 4 drops juniper essential oil

Add evening primrose oil to the grated soap and mix well. Add aloe vera gel and rosewater to soap mixture. Cover and let sit for at least 4 hours. Place mixture in a food processor or blender. Add essential oils 1 drop at a time, mixing well after each addition. Wet hands and form mixture into balls. Let sit on waxed paper to dry and harden. Wrap each soap ball in waxed paper or plastic wrap to store.

CINNAMON-ROSE-OATMEAL SOAP

1 4-ounce bar castile soap, grated
1 Tbsp. sweet almond oil
¼ cup + 2 Tbsp. rosewater
2 Tbsp. ground oatmeal
6 drops cinnamon essential oil
3 drops rosewood essential oil

Mix soap, oil, and rosewater. Let sit for at least 4 hours. Add oatmeal and essential oils. Mix in food processor or blender until well combined. Make into balls and let sit on waxed paper to dry and harden. Wrap each soap ball in waxed paper or plastic wrap to store.

ᏸ BODY AND BATH OILS ᏸ

*M*ake your own! In a popular discount store I saw very small bottles of artificially scented bath oil with dried flowers floating in it for $4 apiece. I know that you can make a superior quality bath oil for much less than that.

There are several kinds of recipes for making bath and body oils. Experiment with these to see which one is the best for you. Any of these can also be used for massage. Remember the old saying "Oil and water don't mix." When putting oil in your bath water it will float on top and coat your body as you get out of the tub. It will also coat the surface of your tub when you let out the water, so be careful that you don't slip. There is a specially treated oil available called Turkey Red Oil that is dispersible in water. You can add this to your bath water and it will mix easily. Essential oils will also float on water and must be mixed with another substance to make them more usable. Two very good ways to use bath and body oils during bath time is to rub the oils on your body before and/or after your bath. That way your skin gets the benefit of the oils and your bath tub doesn't get coated instead of you. For storage and retention of the natural properties of the ingredients, colored glass bottles work the best.

WORK WEARY HANDS OIL

Heavy duty help and protection for hands that are exposed to cold wet conditions. Good for the rest of your body too.

1 Tbsp. castor oil
1 tsp. avocado oil
10 drops evening primrose oil
400 IU Vitamin E
3 drops tea tree essential oil
3 drops chamomile essential oil

Mix all ingredients together. Store in a glass container. Shake before using.

BEST EVER BODY OIL

This is my personal favorite. If I had to choose one skin care product I couldn't live without, it would be this oil. It absorbs easily and keeps all of my body soft, including my hands.

    1 Tbsp. avocado oil
    20 drops jojoba oil
    15 drops carrot seed essential oil
    800 IU Vitamin E
    8 drops rose geranium essential oil
    2 drops lemon essential oil
    2 drops sandalwood essential oil
    2 drops chamomile essential oil

Mix all ingredients except the essential oils. Then, add the carrot seed essential oil and mix. Add the rest of the essential oils and mix well. Store in a glass container.

EXTRA RICH OIL

A luxuriously scented oil that is multipurpose for hands and body.

    1 tsp. avocado oil
    1 tsp. apricot kernel oil
    ¼ tsp. jojoba oil
    ¼ tsp. rosehip seed oil

    ¼ tsp. wheat germ oil
    ¼ tsp. castor oil
    800 IU Vitamin E
    4 drops lavender essential oil
    2 drops cinnamon essential oil
    6 drops ylang-ylang essential oil

Mix all ingredients but essential oils together well. Then, add all of the essential oils and mix. Store in a glass container.

ULTRA HAND OIL

The calendula infused oil adds a healing touch to this all purpose skin oil.

    1 tsp. calendula infused oil
    1 tsp. avocado oil
    800 IU Vitamin E
    6 drops lemon essential oil
    4 drops carrot seed essential oil
    2 drops frankincense essential oil
    2 drops palmarosa essential oil

Mix all ingredients together. Store in a glass bottle.

DISPERSIBLE BATH OIL NO. 1

    1 Tbsp. turkey red oil
    2–4 drops of essential oil, your choice

May use any essential oil for its scent or usefulness to the skin. Check the section on essential oils for a more detailed description of the uses of each one. Mix the ingredients prior to your bath and add to the running water in the tub. You may also mix a larger quantity of this recipe and store in a glass container to use as needed, 1 to 2 Tbsp. at a time.

DISPERSIBLE BATH OIL NO. 2

1 Tbsp. turkey red oil
2 tsp. rosewater

Mix and use in the bath.

NONDISPERSIBLE BATH OIL

This can also be used as a massage oil.
1 Tbsp. base oil (sweet almond or apricot kernel, your choice)
6 drops essential oil, your choice

Do not add more essential oil to base oil than what is stated. This is for the body, not the face. Any higher concentration of essential oils could be irritating to your skin. This could also be mixed in a larger quantity to be used as bath or massage oil as needed. Shake well before using. Store in a dark colored glass container.

ALL PURPOSE BODY OIL

Use before or after bath, and for massage.
1 tsp. wheat germ oil
1 tsp. avocado oil
1 tsp. rosehip seed oil
400 IU Vitamin E
6 drops essential oil, your choice

Mix all ingredients and bottle in glass.

INFUSED OIL

This oil is for external use only. It is a good way to use dried herbs and to transfer the qualities of a specific herb to oil. Olive oil is the best choice of oil to use in this recipe because it has better keeping qualities than some of the others. There two methods of infusing oil.

Method #1:

Take a glass jar and fill to the top with dried or fresh herbs. Fill and cover all the herbs with olive oil, then sit in a sunny window for at least 2 weeks. Strain and refill the jar with more of the same herb. Add the strained oil and top off with more olive oil. Leave in a sunny window for two weeks, then strain and use. Add 800 IU Vitamin E to the oil to help preserve it. Store in a dark glass bottle.

(You could store it in the refrigerator to help prolong the shelf life if you wish.) This makes a good massage oil or it may be used as an ingredient in the making of other products such as hand creams.

Method #2:

½ cup olive oil
3 Tbsp. dried herbs
Place ingredients in a saucepan over very low heat. Allow to warm very gently over the heat for 15 minutes. The oil must not be allowed to get hot enough to spatter or smoke. Watch it very carefully. After 15 minutes remove from heat and strain the mixture. Discard the herbs and store the oil in a dark colored bottle. Add 800 IU Vitamin E to the oil. (You may store the oil in the refrigerator to prolong the shelf life if you wish.) This is a quicker way to obtain your infused oil, but is an appropriate method only when using dried herbs.

∽ FACIAL CARE ∽

*T*he skin on everyone's face is unique. The basic types are dry, normal, oily, sensitive, and blemished. Most people have parts of their face that are one type and parts that are another type. Have an idea of your skin type or types before using any preparation, commercial or homemade. Many of the following are multipurpose, but anything containing alcohol or witch hazel should be avoided or only used rarely on dry skin. Be cautious about what to use on sensitive skin—don't forget to patch test. Don't expect miracles when it comes to removing wrinkles. Facial oils and creams will not remove wrinkles but can help to prevent more wrinkles developing.

CLEANSING GRAINS

These are very fragrant. When you use them, gently scrub your face. Fragile and sensitive skin types should avoid using this product.

¼ cup cornmeal
¼ cup ground oatmeal
½ cup green clay
1 Tbsp. finely ground lavender blossoms
2 Tbsp. finely ground raw sunflower seeds
2 tsp. rosewater
3 drops lavender essential oil
1 drop patchouli essential oil

Add rosewater to clay. Place all ingredients in blender or food processor except essential oils. Process until all ingredients are uniformly coarse. Add essential oils and stir well. Mix 1–2 tsp. with water to make into a paste and gently massage into skin then rinse off.

FACIAL SCRUB

1 Tbsp. finely ground oatmeal
1 Tbsp. dried lavender
blossoms finely ground
1 Tbsp. dried thyme leaves
finely ground
1 Tbsp. finely ground almonds
4 drops lemon essential oil

Use blender, food processor, or grinder to prepare all of the dry ingredients. Mix together in blender or food processor until the mixture is uniformly coarse. Add essential oil and mix well. Store in glass container. Use 1–2 tsp. of mixture with enough water to make a paste and gently scrub face, rinsing when through. Do not use on sensitive or fragile skin. This can also be used as a body scrub.

CLEANSING LOTION

Good middle of the day product. Dry skin types should avoid this as the alcohol and witch hazel would be too drying.

¼ cup distilled water
2½ tsp. witch hazel
1 Tbsp. rubbing alcohol
8 drops of lemon, juniper, or
lavender essential oils

Add essential oil to the alcohol then add the rest of the ingredients. Store in a glass bottle. Shake well before using. Apply with cotton pads.

DRY SKIN CLEANSER

The olive oil is moisturizing, the honey is hydrating and the vinegar helps to maintain the acid mantle!

1 tsp. olive oil
1 tsp. honey
2 tsp. cider vinegar

Mix all ingredients. Apply to face and leave on for 10–15 minutes. Rinse off with tepid water. Finish off by applying rosewater to the skin.

OILY FACE WASH

1 cup distilled water
1 Tbsp. dried thyme
1 Tbsp. dried calendula
blossoms

Put all ingredients in a saucepan. Simmer covered for 10 minutes. Strain, cool, bottle, and refrigerate until ready to use. Do not rinse off. Store up to 3 days.

FACIAL RINSES

Use the herb suited for your skin type. Make an infusion of ¼ cup dried or ½ cup fresh herbs to 2 cups distilled water. Cool, strain, and bottle. Must refrigerate unused portion—do not keep after 3 days. Rinse face with herbal infusion after washing. Do not rinse off. Use during the day as needed as a refresher lotion.

Here are some herbs that are appropriate to different skin types:

sage or yarrow: oily skin

lady's mantle: normal skin

parsley or lemon balm: dry skin

calendula: blemished skin

basil or peppermint: all skin types

fennel seed: mature skin

SKIN FRESHENER

Wakes you up during a long day—makes you feel refreshed!

1 Tbsp. witch hazel

1 Tbsp. rosewater

2 Tbsp. distilled water

1 drop lavender essential oil

Add essential oil to witch hazel. Let sit for 1 hour. Add rosewater and distilled water. Shake well before use. Apply with cotton pads.

BRACING ASTRINGENT

For use on oily skin only.

¼ cup yarrow

⅓ cup pure grain alcohol

Let sit for 2 days, then strain. Add:

2 Tbsp. witch hazel

Shake well before using. Store in the refrigerator. Use in 2 weeks.

TONER

Toners are similar to astringents. They temporarily close your pores and leave your skin feeling tight and refreshed. The lemon juice and rosewater have a softening effect on your skin. This can also be used as an aftershave. Use on normal to oily skin.

2 Tbsp. fresh squeezed and strained lemon juice

2 Tbsp. distilled water

3 Tbsp. rosewater

2 tsp. rubbing alcohol

4 drops rosemary essential oil

Mix all ingredients together. Shake before using. Must be stored in the refrigerator and used within 2 weeks.

MULTIPURPOSE FACIAL CARE

Use as an aftershave, cleanser, and/or toner.

½ cup dried lavender blossoms

1 cup cider vinegar

Place lavender blossoms in cider vinegar in a glass jar and expose to sunlight for 2 weeks. Strain and discard lavender blossoms. The vinegar will be a lovely rosy-lavender color. Use 1 Tbsp. lavender vinegar in 1 Tbsp. water and put on a clean face. Store in the refrigerator. Use within 2 weeks.

ASTRINGENT

This one would be appropriate for normal to oily skin. The essential oils could be changed to more "masculine" ones for an aftershave.

  1 tsp. witch hazel
  3 tsp. rosewater
  1 tsp. cider vinegar
  1 drop orange essential oil
  1 drop juniper essential oil
Mix together all ingredients—let sit 24 hours before using.

OILY SKIN FRESHENER

It smells wonderful, is simple, and makes your skin feel clean and soft—what more could you want?

  1 Tbsp. strained fresh lemon
    juice
  1 Tbsp. distilled water
Mix together and put on a clean face.

FACIAL SPRITZER, 2 WAYS

Last summer our weather was extremely hot. This recipe kept me feeling refreshed after being outside working. Use on oily or normal skin.

First Way:

  ¼ cup pure grain alcohol
  10 drops lemon, lavender or
    rose essential oil
Mix and place in a closed container. Then add 2 cups distilled water and place in a spray bottle. Shake before using. Close eyes before spraying on your face. Use whenever your face needs refreshing.

Second Way:

  1 cup dried lavender blossoms
    or mint or lemon balm
  2 cups distilled water
Combine the two ingredients and simmer 15 minutes over low heat. Let sit covered for 30 minutes, then strain. Add ¼ cup pure grain alcohol. Place in spray bottle. Store in the refrigerator and use within 2 weeks. Shake before using. Close eyes before spraying on face. Use whenever your face needs refreshing.

FACIAL SPRITZER YOUR WAY

  1 Tbsp. witch hazel
  ¾ cup distilled water
  5 drops essential oil, your
    choice

Mix together witch hazel and essential oils. Leave in a closed container overnight. Add distilled water and place in a spray bottle. Shake well before using. Close eyes before spraying your face. Use whenever your face needs refreshing.

FACIAL OIL

This is a light oil that is put on the skin for a protective moisturizing coating. Use this on dry to normal skin.

    1 Tbsp. jojoba oil
    3 drops lavender essential oil
    2 drops rose geranium
        essential oil
    3 drops carrot seed essential
        oil

Mix all ingredients together. Put in glass bottle, preferably dark colored. Put a very thin coating on face. Wipe off excess with cotton pads.

OILY SKIN FACIAL OIL

Yes, even oily skin can have oil applied to it! This recipe has a cleansing quality with these specific essential oils added to it. I use this on my oily skin and it does not make my skin feel too greasy or oily. It is especially protective during the harsh cold winter months.

    1 Tbsp. apricot kernel oil
    400 IU Vitamin E
    3 drops juniper essential oil
    2 drops lemon essential oil
    2 drops bergamot essential oil

Mix all ingredients and store in a dark colored glass container. Shake well before using. Apply a thin coat on the face, and wipe off excess with a cotton pad.

DRY SKIN FACIAL OIL

Good for sensitive and/or mature skin. Use after a bath or shower when your skin is moist and/or at night after facial cleansing.

    1 Tbsp. sweet almond oil
    2 tsp. avocado oil
    ¼ tsp. rosehip seed oil
    800 IU Vitamin E
    5 drops carrot seed essential
        oil
    2 drops sandalwood essential
        oil
    1 drop myrrh essential oil

Mix the above ingredients and place in a dark colored glass bottle. Shake well before using. Apply a thin coat to skin. Wipe off excess with cotton pads.

∽ FACE MASKS ∽

*F*ace masks are not for everyone. If you have very dry skin, do not use face masks with clay because they can be drying. If you have oily or normal skin do not use a mask more than once every one to two weeks. The following masks will be labeled for the appropriate skin type. Always put a mask on a very clean face. Pat your face dry after rinsing off a mask because the skin is too delicate for rougher handling. Also, do not use face masks prior to going out. They can make your face look reddened immediately after use.

LEMON MASK

This one is for oily skin. It feels very tight when drying on your face, but when rinsed off it will make your skin feel smooth.

1 Tbsp. green clay

Strained juice of 1 lemon

Mix together. This will turn into a very foamy substance that can easily be smoothed onto the face and neck. Leave on 20 minutes or until dry. Rinse off with tepid water.

JOJOBA MASK

This is for oily skin.

1 Tbsp. green clay

5 drops jojoba oil

2 drops lavender essential oil

Mix above ingredients with enough water to make spreadable. Put on face and let dry for 20 minutes. Rinse off with tepid water.

BREWER'S YEAST MASK

Brewer's yeast is soothing to skin. The witch hazel is refreshing. Your skin will feel so soft after using this. Good for normal to oily and/or troubled skin.

    1 Tbsp. brewer's yeast

    2 tsp. witch hazel

    1 drop chamomile essential oil

Mix together and add enough water to make spreadable. It will be lumpy, but spread on your face as best as you can. Leave on 15 minutes then rinse with tepid water.

SMOOTHING MASK

Flaxseed forms a gelatinous substance when soaked or boiled in water. Good for any skin type. It does not feel tight when drying.

    2 tsp. flaxseeds

    Just enough water to cover

Let the seeds and water mixture sit until the flaxseed forms gel. If in a hurry, boil the seed and water mixture until the seeds burst and the gel forms. Allow to cool. Spread the gel on the face. Allow to dry and rinse with tepid water.

MATURE OR DRY SKIN MASK

Your face will feel very soft and smell very fragrant afterwards!

    1 Tbsp. brewer's yeast

    1 tsp. crushed fennel seeds

    ½ cup water

Simmer fennel seeds in water for 10 minutes and strain. Allow to cool. Do not keep the fennel seeds in the water any longer, or they will soak up all the water and there will not be enough fluid to make the mixture spreadable. Mix fennel seed infusion with brewer's yeast. Spread on the face, and leave on for 15 minutes. Rinse with tepid water.

CLAY MASK

Good for oily skin. The rosemary essential oil stimulates the circulation and the lavender essential oil is soothing to the skin. Your skin will feel smooth and smell good after using this mask.

    1 Tbsp. fuller's earth

    1 drop lavender essential oil

    1 drop rosemary essential oil

Add the essential oils to the fuller's earth. Add enough water to make the mixture spreadable. Put on your face and allow to dry. Rinse with tepid water.

LADY'S MANTLE MASK

Makes your face feel soft and tingly. Good for normal to slightly oily skin. This mask could also be applied to a face with dry skin if a thin film of sweet almond or apricot kernel oil is applied under the mask.

　　1 Tbsp. brewer's yeast
　　2 tsp. rosewater
　　1 Tbsp. strong infusion lady's
　　　　mantle (Make with 1 Tbsp.
　　　　chopped herb in ⅔ cup
　　　　boiling water and infuse for
　　　　10 minutes.)

Allow herbal infusion to cool. Mix infusion with rosewater. Add brewer's yeast and smooth on face. Leave on for 15 minutes. Rinse off with tepid water.

FENNEL SEED MASK

So fragrant and makes your skin so soft. This one would be fine for mature skin. The oatmeal is good for any skin type.

　　1 Tbsp. honey
　　1 Tbsp. ground oatmeal
　　1 Tbsp. fennel seed infusion
　　　　(Put 2 tsp. crushed fennel
　　　　seed in ⅓ cup boiling water
　　　　and let soak for 15 minutes,
　　　　then strain and use.)

Mix infusion and honey. Add oatmeal and mix well. Smooth on face. Leave on for 15 minutes, then rinse with tepid water.

OATMEAL MASK

Good for sensitive skin.

　　1 Tbsp. ground oatmeal
　　rosewater

Add rosewater by the teaspoonful to the oatmeal until the mixture is spreadable. Spread on the face and leave on until dry. Rinse off with tepid water.

OATMEAL HERBAL MASK

Oatmeal is good for all skin types. Choose a herbal infusion that suits your skin's needs.

　　1 Tbsp. ground oatmeal
　　herbal infusion, your choice
　　　　(Put 3 Tbsp. dried herb in ⅔
　　　　cup boiling water. Simmer
　　　　10–15 minutes, strain, and
　　　　cool.)

Add enough infusion to make a paste. Smooth on face and leave on for 20 minutes. Use the leftover herbal infusion as a lotion on your face after rinsing off the mask.

Infusions to choose from:

Sage or yarrow: astringent, anti-inflammatory, use on oily skin.
Parsley or lemon balm: dry, aging skin.
Chamomile: sensitive skin.
Fennel seed: invigorating for mature skin.
Basil, peppermint, or thyme: all skin types.
Calendula blossoms: troubled skin.

⤳ AFTER SUN CARE ⤳

*D*espite warnings about protecting our skin from the sun, we all know people who without fail get sunburned and come in reddened and miserable. Here are recipes for some sunburn relief measures. These are meant to be used only on skin reddened from the sun, not for blistered skin.

COOL OFF YOUR SKIN SUMMER BATH

¼ cup dried peppermint or ½ cup fresh peppermint
1 cup water
Boil distilled water—add peppermint and simmer for 15 minutes. Strain and allow to cool to lukewarm. Add to tepid bathwater and soak the heat away.

SUNBURN SOAK

Lavender is traditionally the herb for sunburn care.
1 cup apple cider vinegar
10 drops lavender essential oil
Mix the ingredients. Add to tepid bath water. Soak in tub and sponge affected skin.

LAVENDER SUNBURN RINSE

Add 10 drops lavender essential oil to a large bowl of cool water. Dip sponge or soft cloth into water and sponge off affected areas of the skin.

HERBAL SUNBURN RINSE

¼ cup dried calendula blossoms
2 cups distilled water
Boil water, and add calendula blossoms. Simmer for 30 minutes. Strain and allow to cool. Add 2 Tbsp. of infusion to each pint of cool water. Sponge onto sunburned areas. Store infusion in refrigerator for up to 3 days.

LAVENDER-ALOE RELIEF

Two sunburn relievers combined into one cooling combination.

    1 Tbsp. aloe vera gel

    5 drops lavender essential oil

Mix above and apply directly onto sunburned areas.

    Variation: Use lemon essential oil in place of the lavender.

ᴄᴐ HAIR CARE ᴄᴐ

$\mathcal{H}$air texture and the amount of oil in your hair is mainly heredi-
tary, so you have to learn to live with what you have. Shampoo as often as you feel you need it to keep your hair clean. Hair is
composed of dead cells and will not absorb many substances. Hair
thickeners will coat hair with a film that makes it feel thicker with
more body. Oil treatments will coat the hair and will make it less dry.

Many hair care products are expensive. I have bought bottles of
shampoo with "natural" ingredients from hair stylists for $8 a bottle.
For $1.99 I can buy a bottle of baby shampoo, add drops of essential oil
to it and obtain the same results for my hair at a fraction of the cost.

Try to keep hair care simple. Don't get bogged down with a bathroom shelf full of products. If your hair is dry, give it an oil treatment
and use the appropriate herbs and essential oils for dry hair. If it is oily
use herbs and essential oils appropriate for oily hair. Use the lemon or
vinegar rinses to give your hair shine. Try these recipes instead of expensive beauty salon products. You will be pleasantly surprised!

SCALP TREATMENT FOR DRY HAIR

Use this once every one or two weeks.
  1 Tbsp. jojoba oil
  5 drops carrot seed essential oil
Mix above ingredients together.
Work into scalp and shafts of hair
closest to the scalp. Let sit covered
for 1 hour, then shampoo.

OLIVE OIL TREATMENT

*Good for dry hair, use only once a
week. Gives a lovely sheen to the hair.*
  1 Tbsp. olive oil
Gently warm olive oil and apply
to hair and scalp. Cover with towel
for 20 minutes, then wash hair.

CUSTOMIZED SHAMPOO

Choose the essential oil to suit your type of hair. It's easy and just as good as some of the "natural" shampoos on the market.

1 Tbsp. good quality baby shampoo
4 drops essential oil according to your type of hair
Normal hair: patchouli, juniper, rosemary
Oily hair: lemon, bergamot, juniper, rosemary, thyme
Dry hair: carrot seed

Mix essential oils of your choice into the shampoo. Shampoo hair as usual.

CONDITIONING SHAMPOO

D-panthenol is the one vitamin substance that the hair seems to absorb. It strengthens the hair from within and gives it a nice shine, too.

1 Tbsp. good quality baby shampoo
¼ tsp. d-panthenol

Mix the two ingredients together, and shampoo the hair as usual.

Variation: Add 4 drops of essential oil of your choice to the above recipe for added benefits to your hair.

SHAMPOO FOR DRY HAIR

1 Tbsp. good quality baby shampoo
5 drops jojoba oil
4 drops carrot seed essential oil

Mix all of the ingredients together and shampoo hair as usual.

AFTER SHAMPOO HAIR RINSE

I squeeze several lemons and keep the juice in the refrigerator. It keeps for about a week and I then have it available to use for hair or skin. This rinse keeps my hair soft and shiny. Especially recommended for blonds, but could be used on any hair color.

¼ cup fresh squeezed and strained lemon juice
¼ cup water

Mix together and work into freshly washed hair. Keep on hair 10–15 minutes then rinse.

AFTER SHAMPOO RINSE

Good for any hair type.
¼ cup apple cider vinegar
(Can use infused herbal
vinegar, see below.)
¼ cup distilled water
Mix distilled water and vinegar. May keep in the refrigerator for 2 weeks. Work into your hair after shampooing. Leave on for 15 minutes, then rinse.

Variation: Substitute infused herbal vinegar for the plain cider vinegar. Put ½ cup dried herb of your choice into 2 cups of cider vinegar. Warm vinegar in saucepan over low heat. Add herbs. Put in closed glass container and let sit for 2 weeks. Strain and bottle for use.

BROWN HAIR RINSE

Rosemary also has the reputation for strengthening hair.
4 Tbsp. dried rosemary
2 cups distilled water
Simmer together covered for 15 minutes then let sit for 2 hours. Strain and rinse freshly shampooed hair over and over, catching the fluid in a basin to pour over your hair again.

FRAGRANT HAIR OIL

Especially good for oily hair types.
3 drops rosemary essential oil
or lavender essential oil
Apply the essential oil directly to hair midway into drying it. Finish the drying and styling process.

⨯ NAIL CARE ⨯

*F*ingernails can get a lot of abuse from housework, gardening, and other activities. Your cuticles can get torn and ragged too. Wear gloves when your hands are exposed to harsh conditions to help protect your hands and nails from abuse. Some commercial nail hardeners contain formaldehyde which some people are sensitive to, causing damage to nails and cuticles. Try these recipes as a natural alternative to moisturize nails and cuticles.

NAIL AND CUTICLE OIL

Keeping your cuticles lubricated helps to soften them preventing the formation of hangnails.
¼ tsp. jojoba oil
½ tsp. sweet almond oil
400 IU Vitamin E
2 drops carrot seed essential oil
1 drop eucalyptus essential oil
2 drops lemon essential oil
Mix together and rub a very small amount into nails and cuticles twice a day.

CITRUS-ROSEMARY NAIL AND CUTICLE OIL

¼ tsp. wheat germ oil

¼ tsp. rosehip seed oil
3 drops grapefruit essential oil
3 drops lemon essential oil
2 drops rosemary essential oil
Mix all ingredients and place in a dark colored glass jar. Rub a very small amount into cuticles twice daily.

SOFTENING CUTICLE AND NAIL OIL

¼ tsp. avocado oil
20 drops evening primrose oil
5 drops grapefruit essential oil
5 drops carrot seed essential oil
Mix all ingredients and place in a dark colored glass container. Rub a very small amount into nails and cuticles two or three times a day.

∽ FOOT CARE ∽

FOOT POWDER

This is a good product for hard working feet. It really keeps foot odor and moisture down.

  ½ cup arrowroot powder
  2 Tbsp. clay (fuller's earth, kaolin clay, or green clay)
  1 tsp. rubbing alcohol
  8 drops tea tree essential oil
  10 drops peppermint essential oil

Mix arrowroot powder and clay together in a glass container. Add rubbing alcohol and mix. Let sit covered for one hour. Add essential oils and mix well. Let sit covered in a glass container at least 4 hours before using. Place in a shaker container.

CALLOUS TREATMENT

If you don't have any clove essential oil use the rosehip seed oil alone—it is very softening on its own. This recipe can also be used on other roughened areas of the skin such as knees and elbows.

  1 Tbsp. rosehip seed oil
  4 drops clove essential oil

Mix the two ingredients together and store in a glass bottle. Rub a very small amount into callouses and roughened areas twice a day.

☙ BIBLIOGRAPHY ☙

Abehsera, Michel. *The Healing Clay*. New York, NY: Citadel Press, 1990.

Bark, Joseph P., M.D. *Retin A and Other Youth Miracles*. Rocklin, Ca: Prima Publishing and Communication, 1989.

Berwick, Ann. *Holistic Aromatherapy*. St. Paul, Minnesota: Llewellyn Publications, 1994.

Boxer, Arabella, and Phillipa Back. *The Herb Book*. New York, NY: Octopus Books Ltd. 1980.

Bricklin, Mark. *Rodale's Encyclopedia of Natural Home Remedies*. Emmaus, PA: Rodale Press, 1982.

Brumberg, Elaine. *Take Care of Your Skin*. New York, NY: Harper & Row Publishers, 1989.

Buchman, Dian Dincin. *Herbal Medicine*. New York, NY: David McKay Co., Inc., 1979.

Castleman, Michael. *The Healing Herbs*. Emmaus, PA: Rodale Press, 1991.

Cavitch, Susan Miller. *The Natural Soap Book*. Pownal, VT: Storey Publishing, 1995.

Chase, Deborah. *The Medically Based No Nonsense Beauty Book*. New York, NY: Henry Holt & Co., 1989.

Davis, Julie. *Young Skin for Life*. Emmaus, PA: Rodale Press, 1995.

Garland, Sarah. *The Complete Book of Herbs and Spices*. London, England: Frances Lincoln Publishers Ltd., 1979.

Gladstar, Rosemary. *Herbal Healing for Women*. New York, NY: Simon & Schuster, 1993.

Greig, Denise. *The Complete Book of Potpourri and Perfumery*. Kenthurst, New South Wales, Australia: Kangaroo Press, 1992.

Kanner, Catherine. *Beauty from a Country Garden*. Berkley, CA: Ten Speed Press, 1992.

Kowalchik, Claire and William H. Hylton, Editors. *Rodale's Illustrated Encyclopedia of Herbs*. Emmaus, PA: Rodale Press, 1987.

MacKie, Rona M. *Healthy Skin—the Facts*. Oxford, England: Oxford University Press, 1992.

McIntyre, Anne. *The Complete Woman's Herbal*. New York, NY: Henry Holt Co., 1994.

Mills, Simon Y. *Out of the Earth*. New York, NY: Penguin Books, 1991.

Rose, Jeanne. *The Aromatherapy Book*. Berkeley, CA: North Atlantic Books, 1992.

Rose, Jeanne. *Herbs and Things: Jeanne Rose's Herbal*. New York, NY: Perigee Books, 1972.

Ryman, Daniele. *Aromatherapy–The Complete Guide to Plant and Flower Essences for Health and Beauty*. New York, NY: Bantam Books, 1993.

Schoen, Linda Allen, Editor. *The AMA Book of Skin and Hair Care*. Philadelphia, PA: J.P. Lippincott Co., 1976.

Serrentino, Jo. *How Natural Remedies Work*. Point Roberts, WA: Hartley & Marks Inc., 1991.

Stuart, Malcolm, Editor. *The Encyclopedia of Herbs and Herbalism*. New York, NY: Crescent Publishing, 1987.

Tolley, Emelie and Chris Mead. *Gifts from the Herb Garden*. New York, NY: Clarkson Potter Publishers, Inc., 1991.

Worwood, Valerie Ann. *The Complete Book of Essential Oils and Aromatherapy*. San Rafael, Ca: New World Library, 1991.

∽ SOURCES FOR INGREDIENTS ∽

*M*any of the ingredients in these recipes are available in local natural food or herb stores. Check the yellow pages of your phone book to see if any of these stores are near you. If there are no stores in your neighborhood, then use this list of companies to assist you in your search for ingredients.

NOW Natural Foods
available at:
The Fruitful Yield
1-800-469-5552
The quality of NOW products is excellent and so are the prices. I rely on many of their products for my recipes.

Lavender Lane, Inc.
7337 Roseville Road Suite #1
Sacramento, CA 95842
Phone: (916) 334-4400 Fax: (916) 339-0842
You could easily equip yourself with all of the cosmetic ingredients you would need from Lavender Lane. They have all shapes and sizes of glassware for storing your cosmetics, too. Catalog is available.

Herbal Healer Academy, Inc.
HC32, 97-B
Mt. View, AR 72560
Free Brochure/Newsletter (501) 269-4177
This company carries a wide range of books, correspondence lessons, herbs, and other cosmetic supplies. Their catalogue has an interesting variety of items. The Herbal Healer Academy also has a licensed Naturopathic Doctor available for consultations for their lifetime members.

⌒ INDEX ⌒